The Women's Health Companion
Self Help Nutrition Guide & Cookbook

The Women's Health Companion

Self Help Nutrition Guide & Cookbook

Susan M. Lark, M.D.

CELESTIAL ARTS
BERKELEY, CALIFORNIA

NOTE: The information in this book is meant to complement the advice and guidance of your physician, not replace it. It is very important that women who have medical problems be evaluated by a physician. If you are under the care of a physician, you should discuss any major changes in your regimen with him or her. Because this is a book and not a medical consultation, keep in mind that the information presented here may not apply in your particular case. In view of individual medical requirements, new research, and government regulations, it is the responsibility of the reader to validate health practices and treatment with a physician or health service.

Celestial Arts Publishing
P. O. Box 7123
Berkeley, CA 94707

Library of Congress-in-Publication Data

Lark, Susan M., 1945-
      The woman's health companion: self help nutrition guide
and cookbook/ Susan Lark.
          p. cm.
      Includes bibliographical references and index.
      ISBN 0-89087-797-1
       1. Women—Nutrition. 2. Generative organs, Female—Diseases—
Diet therapy. 3. Women—Diseases—Diet therapy. I. Title.
      RA778.L314 1994   94-18485
      613.2'082—dc20   CIP

Cover by Ken Scott
Illustrations © 1995 by Lisa Tranter Sibony
Text design by Sarah Levin

Printed in the United States
First Paper Printing, 1996

1 2 3 4 5 / 00 99 98 97 96

To my wonderful husband Jim and
my darling daughter Rebecca

To the health and well-being of all women

Contents

Why I Wrote This Book

As a physician specializing in women's health care and preventive medicine for nearly twenty years, I have always emphasized nutrition as an important part of a health program. When women make the transition from poor dietary habits and poor health, to good nutrition and vital health, many find that following specific guidelines helps them with this process. With this in mind, I began to give my patients basic nutritional education and information, and sometimes even menus, meal plans, and recipes. Many of these women say these tools make their meal planning and preparation easier and enhance the enjoyment they derive, and their families derive, from more healthful meals.

Often, my patients ask me to recommend a cookbook for women's special nutritional needs—a cookbook that would also help them prepare meals that would be equally beneficial for the entire family. Unfortunately, no such cookbook exists, and none even gives women the in-depth nutritional information to they need to make dietary choices as educated consumers. To fill this gap, and to provide women with these resources, I have written this book.

Using Nutrition to Help Myself

I first became aware of the importance of nutrition during my first year of postgraduate training after medical school. Since my early teenage years, I suffered from two very common female complaints—menstrual cramps and PMS. Throughout my teens and twenties I found very few treatment options available to me for cramps except aspirin, hot water bottles, and lying in bed for hours in pain, hoping it would stop. Since I also suffered from PMS, my menstrual cramps were preceded by days of anxiety, irritability, bloating, and food cravings. It is no wonder that I regarded each period with apprehension. Very little information was available on self-care treatments at that time. Although my parents were caring, I received absolutely no information from them on the importance of nutrition and exercise in preventing and relieving my symptoms.

My PMS and menstrual cramp symptoms continued to be quite severe throughout college and medical school. As a doctor-in-training, I had access to the best medical care. I tried every medication possible that might help me—pain pills, muscle relaxants, and antispasmodics—but these only relieved my symptoms temporarily. I still remember when I was a medical student and episodes of menstrual cramps were severe enough to compel me to leave the hospital ward. I would go to the medical students' on-call room and suffer through the agony of viselike cramps.

My situation changed during my internship year. I was doing my specialty training in obstetrics and gynecology and spent quite a bit of time reading the new medical research in this field. By chance, I spotted an article in an obstetrics and gynecology journal on the use of nutrition to treat breast cysts. I had never been exposed to the concept of nutrition as therapy before. In fact, it had never occurred to me that what I ate could affect my state of health. I was intrigued by the article, which described the successful treatment of breast lumps with the use of vitamins. I began spending time in the medical library searching for information on the treatment of menstrual disorder through nutrition.

During the next few years, I began to test a simple program on myself. I made many dietary changes and cut out sugar, fat, and caffeine, which had been the mainstay of my diet. As a medical student, I had depended on "fast foods" such as cola drinks, coffee, sweet rolls, and ham sandwiches to help me stay awake and provide a quick source of energy during busy late nights taking care of patients. I started cutting down on my junk food intake and began eating more whole grains, fresh vegetables, and fruits. I started a vitamin and mineral program that I developed based on my research in nutritional medicine.

I was amazed at the results. My symptoms, which had plagued me for years, began to diminish each month. My quality of life improved dramatically as my symptoms receded. I felt better than I had in my entire life. With a healthier diet, my symptoms disappeared completely and never came back.

For the past two decades, my menstrual periods have been painless and symptom-free. I am now turning fifty years old and have had many years of periods that haven't interfered with my life. In fact, they are so comfortable that I never know when they are going to start, except for the fact that I keep a menstrual calendar. With the continued practice of good nutritional habits, I am planning to have an equally comfortable menopause when that phase of life begins.

How to Use This Book

This book was written to provide complete information about all aspects of nutrition for women. The information has been divided into four sections: Part I: Foods to Eat and Foods to Avoid; Part II: Vitamins, Minerals, and Herbs for Female Health Problems; Part III: Food Preparation and the Healthy Kitchen; and Part IV: Menus and Recipes.

Some of the ingredients in recipes may be unfamiliar to you, for example products that replace "high-stress" ingredients such as sugar, salt, cream, and butter. All of these products are readily available in most stores or by mail order. I enjoy their excellent flavor and high nutrient quality. Why not approach new, unfamiliar food with the anticipation of pleasure and enjoyment, much the way you do when trying a new restaurant?

I have been delighted over the years with the benefits that my dietary recommendations produce for my patients, and often their families. Many women have told me that their husbands or significant others have lost weight; their blood pressure and cholesterol levels have gone down; their immune functions have improved with fewer colds, flus, and allergies; and even their arthritis joint pains have disappeared. I have also been told by many patients that their children are much healthier and have fewer school absences for colds and other infections.

The recipes in this book are quick, simple, and easy to prepare. I have found that anything too complicated doesn't work for me or for most other women. Most women lead full, active lives and don't have the time to spend endless hours in the kitchen. Don't be afraid to modify the recipes if you want to change the proportions and flavors to suit your taste. I do this myself when I read cookbooks and want to adapt the dishes to the tastes of my own family.

Best of all, these recipes are delicious and satisfying as well as highly nutritious. All of the recipes have been carefully planned and tested to include the nutrients most needed for your health as well as the flavor and enjoyment of your meals. I hope that you enjoy them and that they provide you and your family with good health and delicious dining.

Part I

Foods to Eat
and
Foods to Avoid

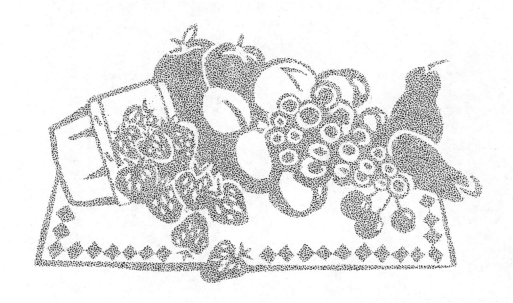

Foods to Eat for Good Health

An optimum diet containing an abundance of high-nutrient, low-stress foods is the basis for good health, energy, and a sense of well-being. During nearly two decades of working with thousands of women patients, I have been continually impressed by the health benefits that good nutritional habits provide. As a result, I spend a great deal of time counseling my patients nutritionally. It is important to me that women have the knowledge and information that they need to effectively plan and prepare their own meals.

Chapter 1 discusses the foods that we need to eat to assure good health: whole grains, legumes, raw seeds and nuts, fish, poultry, fruits, vegetables, sweeteners, herbs and spices, and water. This chapter covers not only the nutrient benefits of these foods and how best to include them, but also their role in relieving and preventing a variety of female health problems and other health issues. Be sure to incorporate these foods abundantly in your daily diet while enjoying their good flavors and textures.

Whole Grains

Whole grains are the seeds of various grasses and are often referred to as "cereals." They have been the mainstay of the human diet for thousands of years, as our body's main source of fuel and energy. While the grains consumed in different societies vary greatly—wheat in the United States, rice in the Orient—they provide the backbone for all diets. In fact, a meal without grain often feels incomplete and somehow lacking.

Whole grains are almost complete meals within themselves, containing fiber, protein, carbohydrates, fats, vitamins such as B and E complexes, and many minerals like calcium, magnesium, potassium, iron, copper, and manganese. There are three main parts to each kernel of grain: the **endosperm**, or central core, which is about 80 percent of the entire kernel; the **germ**, which comprises about 3 percent; and the **bran**, which encompasses 15 percent of the kernel. Whole grain products contain all three parts of the grain and have a high concentration of nutrients. However, when grain is refined in milling to produce white flour products, the germ and bran are removed, leaving only the endosperm. As a result, most of the essential nutrients of the grain are removed, leaving a devitalized product.

The nutrients of whole grains help promote good overall health. They also have a tremendous effect on relieving the symptoms and reducing the risk of a wide variety of female-related health problems. Whole grains have a very potent effect on regulating estrogen levels in the body, through their high levels of phytoestrogens (natural plant estrogens), their fiber content, and their high levels of vitamin B complex and vitamin E.

Many whole grains are excellent sources of phytoestrogens. Whole grains contain lignans, cellulose-like materials that provide structure to plants. Lignans have been found to be weakly

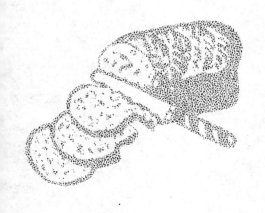

estrogenic and can bind to the estrogen receptors of cells. As a result, they can provide additional nutritional support to menopausal women deficient in this hormone. In addition, certain plants like buckwheat are excellent sources of the bioflavonoid rutin. Like lignans, many bioflavonoids are estrogenic and can help to regulate the effects of our own body's estrogen on sensitive target tissue like the breast and uterus. Rutin is particularly helpful in its ability to strengthen capillaries and reduce heavy menstrual bleeding in transitioning menopausal women. Studies attest to this. Bioflavonoids have been used, along with vitamin C, to reduce heavy bleeding in transitioning menopausal women and women with bleeding due to fibroid tumors and spontaneous abortions. In fact, an early study done at the University of Tennessee Medical School in 1956 found that the bioflavonoid-vitamin C combination allowed 78 percent of high-risk women to carry their pregnancies to full term.

The high-fiber content of whole grains benefits women during their active reproductive years as well as menopausal women. Fiber binds to estrogen in the intestinal tract and removes it from the body through the bowel movements, thus helping to regulate estrogen levels. This process, called the enterohepatic circulation of estrogen, occurs as follows: estrogen circulates in the blood throughout the body and passes through the liver; the liver then metabolizes it from its more potent forms, estradiol and estrone, to a more chemically inactive and weaker form, estriol. When the liver is healthy this occurs efficiently. The estrogen metabolites are then secreted into the bile and from there, into the digestive tract.

With a high-fat, low-fiber diet, the bacteria in the intestinal tract act on these estrogen products, allowing reabsorption of the estrogen back into the body. This increases the blood levels of estrone, the primary type of estrogen produced by the body after menopause, and estradiol, the type of estrogen produced by the ovaries during the active reproductive years. As a result, the levels of these two estrogens rise higher than estriol, their primary breakdown product. When this occurs, the patient is said to have an "unhealthy estrogen profile." Research has shown that estradiol and estrone, as more chemically active and potent forms of estrogen, may predispose women towards developing heavy menstrual bleeding, fibroid tumors, PMS, and even breast cancer while estriol, a much weaker form of estrogen, may reduce the risk and severity of these problems. Thus, a high-fiber, low-fat diet may help regulate not only the estrogen levels but also the types of estrogen circulating throughout a woman's body. In fact, other studies from Tufts University Medical School have shown that vegetarian women excrete two to three times more estrogen in their bowel movements than do women eating the typical high-fat, low-fiber diet.

Whole grains also regulate hormonal levels due to their high levels of vitamin B and vitamin E, which have a beneficial effect on both the liver and the ovaries. In 1942, a researcher named Biskind found that B vitamin deficiency hindered the liver's ability to metabolize estrogen levels in both animal and human test subjects. The addition of B vitamin supplementation to the diet of women suffering from PMS, heavy menstrual bleeding, and fibrocystic breast disease helped to decrease the severity of their symptoms. Studies conducted at UCLA Medical School during the 1980s found that taking a specific B vitamin, pyridoxine B_6, helped to relieve symptoms of menstrual cramps and PMS.

Research also conducted during the 1980s at Johns Hopkins University Medical Center similarly found, in several placebo-controlled studies, that vitamin E is useful in reducing many PMS symptoms, as well as fibrocystic breast discomfort. Other studies have found that vitamin E supplementation reduced menopause-related hot flashes, fatigue, and mood swings in 66 to 85 percent of the women tested, depending on the study. One additional study noted a decrease in the symptoms of vaginal atrophy in 50 percent of the postmenopausal women volunteers.

Besides regulating estrogen levels, the high-fiber content of whole grains binds to cholesterol, aiding its excretion from the body through the digestive tract. This helps lower blood cholesterol levels, reducing the risk of heart attacks in post-menopausal women. The fiber in grain is very helpful in relieving constipation, as well as in preventing other diseases of the digestive tract such as diverticulitis and hiatal hernia. It may also have a protective effect against colon cancer, another disease found commonly in those who eat a high-fat, low-fiber diet.

Whole grains are excellent sources of carbohydrates, which are capable of stabilizing blood sugar and helping to eliminate sugar cravings. They help prevent or control diabetes mellitus, a dangerous disease that predisposes people toward heart disease, blood vessel problems, infections, and blindness. Fifty percent of our population above the age of sixty have blood sugar abnormalities, due in great part to the tremendous amount of highly sugared foods and sweets Americans eat. Whole grains, with their natural sweetness, can satisfy much of this craving in a healthful way.

In addition, whole grains are an excellent source of complete protein when combined in a meal with legumes. Grains are low in the essential amino acid lysine, while legumes are low in methionine. When eaten in combination, they create a high-quality, complete protein. Good examples of grain/legume meals include whole grain bread with a bowl of bean soup, or pasta salad with kidney beans or garbanzos.

Whole grains also contain many vital nutrients for menopausal women. Grains are excellent sources of magnesium and calcium. Both of these minerals are necessary for maintaining healthy bones and relaxing muscle tension. Grains are also high in potassium. Potassium has a diuretic effect on the body's tissues and helps reduce bloating, which can be a problem for premenstrual and postmenopausal women.

While consuming whole grains has many health benefits, some women may find that they are allergic to or intolerant of wheat. Most women are surprised by this discovery, since wheat is one of the staples of our culture and is eaten by most people at almost every meal. However, wheat contains a protein called gluten, which is highly allergenic and difficult for the body to break down, absorb, and assimilate. Women with wheat intolerance are prone to fatigue, depression, bloating, intestinal gas, and bowel changes.

In my clinical experience, when women are nutritionally sensitive, wheat consumption can often worsen emotional symptoms and lower energy levels. I have observed how wheat (along with other foods) can trigger emotional symptoms and fatigue in PMS patients, especially during the week or two before the onset of menses. Many menopausal women tolerate wheat poorly because their digestive tracts are beginning to show the wear and tear of aging and don't produce enough enzymes to break down wheat easily.

Women with allergies often find that wheat intensifies nasal and sinus congestion, as well as fatigue. I also find that women with poor resistance and a tendency toward infections may need to eliminate wheat from their diets to boost their immune systems. Since wheat is leavened with yeast, it should also be avoided by women with candida.

If you suffer from any of these conditions, you should probably eliminate wheat from your diet for at least one to three months. Oats and rye, which also contain gluten, should be eliminated initially along with wheat if your symptoms are severe. Many highly allergic or severely upset and fatigued women don't even handle corn or rice well. Although corn and rice do not contain gluten, most women eat them so frequently that they build up an intolerance to them during times of fatigue.

I have found over the years that the least stressful grain for women with severe allergies, PMS symptoms, and poor digestive function is buckwheat. This is probably because it is not commonly eaten in our culture, so most women never develop an intolerance to it. Also, it is not in the same plant family as wheat and other grains. (Buckwheat is actually the fruitlike structure of the plant rather than a grass.) Other infrequently used grains such as wild rice, quinoa, and amaranth should be tried as well. These are available in health food stores in pastas and cereals. As women with gluten intolerance (and even grain intolerance) start to regain their health, they can slowly increase their grain intake, adding other grains. Wheat intake, however, should still be limited to small quantities, with other alternative grains emphasized instead. In addition, rotating a variety of nongluten grains in the diet can be very helpful. Corn and rice can replace wheat. Often you can find pasta and noodles, as well as flour for baking, made from these grains. Use corn tortillas instead of wheat.

Whole grass and whole grain flours can be prepared in a variety of ways, including whole grain cereals, breads, crackers, pancakes, waffles, and pastas. They can also be sprouted and eaten raw. A wide variety of these grains and products are available both in supermarkets and natural food stores.

Hot Cereals. Local health food stores sell a wide range of excellent grain cereals. If you prefer hot cereals, look for cream of rye, cream of buckwheat, whole grain oatmeal, and seven- or four-grain cereals (without wheat). Choose brands with no added sugar. If there is no health food store near you, most supermarkets will have adequate products and are even beginning to carry bulk cereals in bins. I highly recommend Quaker whole oatmeal (not the quick-cooking refined product). Many of the "natural cereals" from the large companies are highly refined or highly sugared, so read labels carefully.

Cold Cereals. Cold cereals are also available in a wide variety of grains. In health food stores, look for puffed rice, corn, millet, and unsweetened granola. At supermarkets, look for products labeled "whole grain." Cheerios and All-Bran cereals, among others, are good choices. Avoid cold cereals with added sugar.

I suggest moistening your cereal with nondairy milk: soy milk, nut milk, or the excellent new potato-based milks. Many of these are fortified with calcium, contain no saturated fat, and are digested relatively easily. Nondairy milk enables you to avoid the negative effect of dairy products on your mood and energy level. (See Chapter 2 for more information on the pitfalls of dairy products.) Some women enjoy eating cold cereals dry or with a small amount of apple juice. For sweeteners, try fructose or maple syrup. They are very concentrated in flavor, so a little goes a long way.

Muffins, Breads, and Crackers. A wide variety of whole grains can be found in the breads, muffins, and crackers now available in health food stores and supermarkets. There are also simple recipes available if you wish to prepare baked goods, such as oat muffins with extra oat bran, rye muffins, or corn bread. Rice cakes are readily available at health food stores and now increasingly stocked at neighborhood supermarkets. You can also find sprouted wheat and wheat-free bread in health food stores and some supermarkets. Muffins, bread, and crackers can be eaten with applesauce, nut butter, fruit, or preserves. Try to avoid cow's milk butter, which is high in saturated fat.

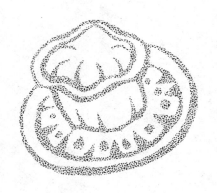

Pancakes and Waffles. Besides wheat flour, you can make pancakes with buckwheat, rice flour, or triticale. Concentrated sweeteners such as maple syrup, honey, and applesauce can be used in small amounts. Try to avoid topping pancakes and waffles with excess butter or whipped cream. This changes them from healthful food to unhealthy food laden with fat, sugar, and calories.

Pasta. Pasta made of buckwheat, rice, corn, or soy is readily available in health food and ethnic food stores. These non-wheat pastas add a wide variety of colors and flavors to the wheat-based white flour pasta found in supermarkets. They are easy to digest for women who have digestive symptoms and bloating with menstruation.

Sprouts. Many people like the nutty, delicious flavor of raw sprouts. Several grains, as well as beans and peas, can be sprouted easily at home with sprouting jars (available at natural food stores). Sprouting softens the grains so that they can be eaten without cooking. High in vitamins and minerals, sprouts can be added to salads, casseroles, and other entrees to boost the nutritional value of these foods.

Cooked grains. Grains are very easy to cook at home and should be eaten as an integral part of most meals. Rice, millet, and other grains are prepared simply by boiling water, adding grain, and letting them cook over low heat until the water has been absorbed and the grains are light and fluffy in texture. Some women prefer the convenience of a rice steamer, which can prepare grains in larger quantities. Grains store for several days in the refrigerator in a jar or plastic container; they can then be reheated and added to dishes. Rice is best reheated by placing it over a double boiler or in a steamer and cooking it for three to five minutes.

If you have a wheat intolerance, you can still make your own baked goods. Simply use rice flour and enjoy its mild flavor. For more intensely flavored baked goods, experiment with combining milder flavored flour with more intensely flavored ones like rye flour.

Types of Grains (or Grainlike) Foods

Amaranth	Millet	Spelt
Barley	Oats	Triticale
Buckwheat	Quinoa	Wheat
Corn	Rice	Wild rice
Kamut	Rye	

Legumes (Beans and Peas)

Legumes are highly recommended foods for women. There are dozens of members of the legume family, including garbanzo beans, kidney beans, lima beans, black beans, lentils, pinto beans, split peas, green peas, soybeans, and many others. All legumes are excellent sources of protein, particularly when combined with whole grains. When consumed together, legumes and grains provide a full range of essential amino acids, the building blocks of protein. Legumes tend to be low in the amino acid methionine, while whole grains are low in lysine. Thus, the two foods complement one another when eaten at the same meal. (Good examples of grain and legume combinations are meals such as beans and rice, or cornbread and split pea soup.) Legumes provide an important and easily utilized source of protein and can be used as a substitute for meat.

Legumes are also an excellent source of both soluble and insoluble types of fiber. The fiber content of beans enables the digestive system to break them down easily and absorb their nutrients, such as protein and carbohydrates, in a slower manner. This has many health benefits. The slow digestion of legume-based carbohydrates can help regulate the blood sugar level. As a result, they are a highly beneficial food for women with blood sugar imbalances or diabetes. The fiber, itself, can help normalize bowel function and lower cholesterol levels by promoting excretion of cholesterol through the bowel movements. Legumes with the highest fiber content are black beans, garbanzo beans, mung beans, pinto beans, split peas, lentils, and navy beans.

Legumes are valuable sources of many other nutrients needed by menopausal women, including calcium, magnesium, and potassium. Calcium and magnesium build strong bones, and potassium helps regulate the heartbeat. All three minerals are important in maintaining healthy muscle tone, combating fatigue, controlling mood swings, and promoting endurance and stamina. Legumes are also very high in iron and vitamin B complex. Sufficient iron intake is particularly important for teenage girls, pregnant women, and women with bleeding problems who are transitioning into menopause. Vitamin B complex is also essential for health, helping the liver regulate estrogen levels. (The liver metabolizes estrogen so that it can be excreted efficiently from the body.)

Because they are an excellent food source of vitamin B_6, legumes, eaten regularly, can help to relieve and prevent PMS symptoms and menstrual cramps. Studies done at UCLA Medical School during the 1980s found vitamin B_6 to be useful for both conditions.

Not only do legumes, in general, have many health benefits for all women, but soybean-based products in particular can actually help reduce and prevent menopause symptoms. Soybeans are filled with natural plant estrogens (or phytoestrogens) called bioflavonoids. Certain bioflavonoids are weak estrogens, having 1/50,000 the potency of a dose of synthetic estrogen. As weak estrogens, these compounds bind to estrogen receptors and act as a substitute form of estrogen in the body. They compete with the more potent estrogens made by a woman's body for these cell receptor sites. As a result, bioflavonoids can help to regulate estrogen levels.

High estrogen levels can worsen female problems like heavy menstrual flow, PMS, fibroid tumors of the uterus, endometriosis, and fibrocystic breast lumps. A soy-based diet can decrease the severity of these problems by reducing the toxic effects of the more potent estrogens on estrogen-sensitive tissues like the breast and uterus.

After menopause, when estrogen levels can become deficient, dietary sources of estrogen such as soy can provide much-needed hormonal support for the body. In fact, a diet high in bioflavonoid-rich soybeans can actually reduce the incidence of menopause symptoms. In Japan, where soybeans are a staple food, only 10 to 15 percent of the women experience menopause symptoms. By contrast, 80 to 85 percent of women in the United States, Canada, and Europe who eat a traditional Western diet experience menopausal symptoms.

One study reported in the *British Medical Journal* in 1990 examined how shifting the diet towards phytoestrogen-containing foods can change certain menopause indicators. By this study, 25 menopausal women (average age fifty-nine) were asked to supplement their normal diet with phytoestrogen-containing foods like soy flour, flax seed oil, and red clover sprouts. The women consumed these foods over a six-week period, each food for two weeks at a time. Smears of the vaginal wall were taken every week to see if the addition of estrogen-containing plant foods would cause a beneficial hormonal effect on the vagina. (Typically, the vaginal mucosa thins out and becomes more prone to trauma and infections as the estrogen level drops with menopause.) Interestingly, the vaginal mucosa did respond significantly to the intake of soy flour and flax oil (not to the red clover sprouts) but returned to its previous state eight weeks after these foods were discontinued and the women went back to their normal diets. Studies have also shown the benefit of soybeans in reducing hot flashes.

Other research studies have measured phytoestrogen excretion, comparing groups with a diet rich in soy and other phytoestrogens to groups eating the typical Western omnivorous diet. One study, published in 1991, showed that men, women, and children in Japan and America who ate a diet high in soy foods like tofu, boiled soybeans, and miso excreted 100 to 1000 times more beneficial bioflavonoids in their urine than women in Finland and the United States who ate a meat- and dairy-based diet. In fact, bioflavonoid content tends to be 80 percent lower in the typical American or European meat- and dairy-based diet, than it is in a vegetarian-based diet.

The bioflavonoids found in soybeans have the added benefit of being anticarcinogenic. Research has linked a high intake of soybean-based foods to the lower incidence of breast cancer and lower mortality from prostate cancer among Japanese women and men, respectively. Other clinical studies have found that soy helps to lower cholesterol levels, thereby helping to reduce the incidence of heart attacks.

Soy is available in many forms in the United States. Tofu, an inexpensive, bland, curdlike soy product, can be found in most supermarkets and health food stores. Tofu will take on the flavor of any food that you cook it with, which makes it an ideal source of protein and essential fatty acids that you can add to soups, stir-fries, casseroles, and other dishes. Tempeh is a cultured soy product made of the whole soybean. Besides being a good source of protein, it contains vitamin B_{12}, a nutrient needed for the production of healthy blood cells and nerve function. Purely vegetarian diets are often deficient in vitamin B_{12}. Thus, adding tempeh can be helpful.

Soy flour makes a tasty substitute for white flour in muffins, breads, pasta, cookies, and other baked goods. It is an excellent source of bioflavonoids. Soy vegetable protein, with its nutty flavor, can be used as a beef substitute in tacos, chili, burritos, and other dishes.

One of the most interesting uses of soy is as a dairy substitute. Any product that comes from a cow is now available in a soy-based version. This includes soy milk cheese, sour cream, yogurt, cream cheese, and ice cream-like desserts. Many of these products are surprisingly good-tasting and have a pleasing texture. In fact, I find several brands of soy yogurt, sour cream, and cream cheese to be almost indistinguishable from their dairy counterparts. Although the soy cheeses generally tend not to be as tasty or textured, Soyco and Soymage are delicious. Soy-based meat such as hot dogs, burgers, and other substitute meat products can be very tasty too. Be sure to look at the label of each product to make sure that it is not too high in either salt or fat.

Besides soy, many other legumes are available in ready-to-use products. In the frozen food section of your local health food store, you'll find low-fat and low-salt versions of many ethnic dishes, such as Indian curries with lentils and Mexican entrées with black or kidney beans. In delicatessens, look for hummus, a nutritious Middle Eastern dip made from garbanzo beans. Even in supermarkets, you can find numerous other bean-based entrées, soups, and salads.

To prepare your favorite dishes at home, you can buy a variety of canned, frozen, and bottled legumes. Many types of legumes are available with low or no added salt; it is important, however, to check the label of the can or carton to make sure advertising claims are true. Health food stores also sell several brands of canned beans grown without pesticides or herbicides, an important consideration for women who are chemically sensitive. All legumes combine well with a wide variety of other foods. Include them often to add protein to your home-made soups, salads, casseroles, stir-fries, dips, and other dishes.

Many women feel discouraged from cooking beans and grains because of their lengthy preparation time. Here is a method to speed up cooking time for beans:

Bring water to a boil (three cups of water for every cup of beans). Add the beans to the boiling water and cook for two minutes. Remove from heat, partially cover pan, and let beans cook for one hour. Go about your business or chores during this time as the beans continue to cook. After one hour, drain and rise with cold water and then freeze. When you are ready to use the beans for a meal, thaw them quickly under running water. Boil five cups of water in a pot for every cup of beans. Add the beans. Lower the heat and cook for 30 to 50 minutes. The beans will be ready to eat.

Some women find that gas is a problem when they eat beans. You can minimize gas by taking digestive enzymes and eating beans in small quantities. Also, because legumes contain high levels of protein, they may be difficult to digest at first for women with severe fatigue or digestive problems. For easier digestibility, I recommend beginning with green beans, green peas, split peas, lentils, lima beans, fresh sprouts, and tofu (if you handle soy products well). As your energy level improves, add delicious legumes such as black beans, pinto beans, kidney beans, and chickpeas.

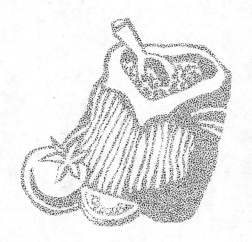

Common Legumes

Adzuki beans	Green beans	Navy beans
Black beans (turtle beans)	Green peas	Pinto beans
	Kidney beans	Red beans
Black-eyed peas	Lentils	Snow peas

Cranberry beans	Lima beans	Soybeans
Garbanzo beans	Mung beans	Split peas
Great Northern beans		

Seeds and Nuts

Both seeds and nuts contain the embryo that allows plants to procreate future generations. The seed is the ripened ovule of a flowering plant. Within the protective coat of the seed lies the embryo and all the stored food that it needs to develop into a new plant. Nuts are single-seeded fruits of various trees and shrubs. They consist of a kernel sealed within a hard, leathery shell.

Many seeds and nuts are edible; these form an important part of the human diet and the diet of many other animals. They have a variety of textures and flavors. Eaten whole, seeds and nuts are sources of many important nutrients, including healthful polyunsaturated fats; protein; B complex vitamins; vitamins A, D, and E; and many minerals such as calcium, potassium, magnesium, iron, copper, zinc, and phosphorous. Seeds and nuts are also important sources of many oils used in cooking and food preparation.

The healthy essential oils found in many seeds and nuts—linoleic acid and linolenic acid—are extremely beneficial for women of all ages. Linoleic acid, part of the Omega-6 family of fatty acids, is primarily found in raw seeds and nuts. Good sources include flax seeds, pumpkin seeds, sesame seeds, sunflower seeds, and walnuts. The other essential fatty acid, linolenic acid, is a member of the Omega-3 family and is primarily found in plant sources such as flax seeds, soy, pumpkin seeds, walnuts, and green leafy vegetables as well as certain fish like salmon, trout and mackerel. Both essential fatty acids must be derived from dietary sources, as the body cannot manufacture them.

The body burns the essential fatty acids not for energy, but for special functions necessary for good health and survival. Our skin is filled with fatty acids that, along with estrogen, provide moisture, softness, and smooth texture. When estrogen levels decline with menopause, we can continue to provide moisture to the skin, vagina, and bladder mucosa by increasing levels of fatty acid-containing foods. Flax seed oil is particularly good for dry skin since it contains high levels of both fatty acids. In addition, fatty acids are a main structural component of all cell membranes and are found in high levels in such important tissues as the brain and nerve cells, adrenal gland, retina, and inner ear.

Besides relieving tissue dryness, essential fatty acids are needed by the body as precursors for the production of important hormone-like chemicals called prostaglandins. Body tissues manufacture over thirty types of prostaglandins. The proper balance of prostaglandins can play a major role in relieving and preventing many diseases that occur predominantly in the postmenopausal period.

The series one prostaglandins are manufactured by the body from linoleic acid. These prostaglandins have many beneficial effects. One member of the series, called prostaglandin E, or PGE, is particularly helpful for women during their active reproductive years. PGE helps to regulate and relax uterine tone as well as the tension of other muscles in the body. As a result, it protects against developing menstrual cramps. PGE also regulates blood circulation and the diameter of the blood vessels, thus helping to prevent PMS tension headaches. It plays a role in optimizing fluid balance, thereby reducing PMS-related bloating, fluid retention, and breast tenderness. In addition, women need adequate levels of this important prostaglandin to prevent PMS-related emotional upset, allergies, and lack of resistance to infection.

Menopausal women also need PGE to achieve and maintain optimal health. PGE keeps the platelets, a component of blood, from sticking or clumping together. This reduces the likelihood of heart attacks and strokes by preventing clotting of the blood and obstruction of the blood vessels. Since the incidence of heart attacks increases tenfold between the ages of fifty-five and sixty-five, PGE can benefit women in this age group greatly. In addition, PGE reduces inflammation, and thus the symptoms of arthritis. Many women date the onset of arthritis symptoms after menopause. PGE also stimulates immune function and helps insulin to function effectively. Obviously, a diet high in raw seeds and nuts, promoting series one prostaglandin production, is beneficial to menopausal women.

Besides the many benefits of seed-and-nut derived oils, flax oil, in particular, has one other special property. The oil is estrogenic and can attach itself to the estrogen receptors in the cells. This can provide a very important extra dietary source of estrogen for postmenopausal women who are showing signs of hormone deficiency.

Besides their high content of essential oils, seeds and nuts are excellent sources of protein. In fact, many commonly eaten seeds such as pumpkin, sesame, and sunflower contain significantly more protein than grains. For example, sesame seeds are 20 percent protein, while sunflower seeds are 25 percent protein. Nuts are similarly rich sources of protein, with almonds and walnuts each containing 20 percent. The protein content of hazelnuts and pecans is somewhat less, at 15 and 10 percent, respectively. When combined with other sources of vegetable protein, seeds and nuts can help to round out and complete a meal.

Seed and nuts are excellent sources of B-complex vitamins and vitamin E, both of which are important antistress factors for women with anxiety, mood swings, and fatigue. These nutrients also help regulate hormonal balance and relieve PMS and menopausal symptoms.

Like vegetables, seeds and nuts are very high in the essential minerals needed by all women such as magnesium, calcium, and potassium. Particularly beneficial are sesame seeds (a rich source of calcium), sunflower seeds, pistachios, pecans, and almonds. However, one drawback of eating too many seeds is their phosphorus content, which can throw off calcium balance. Thus, ancillary sources of calcium need to be included in the diet. (Nuts are not such a problem in this regard.) Another drawback is that seeds and nuts are also very high in calories and should be eaten in moderate amounts.

The oils in all seeds and nuts are highly perishable, so avoid exposing them to light, heat, and oxygen. I recommend refrigerating all shelled seeds and nuts, as well as their oils, to prevent rancidity. Try to eat them raw, and, if you can, shell them yourself. The intact shell keeps the nuts fresh and delicious. Once you buy them, keep them in a tightly covered container away from the hot stove until you are ready to eat them. Eating them raw and unsalted gives you the benefit of their essential fatty acids, and you'll also avoid the negative effects of too much salt. I've also found raw seeds and nuts to be more easily digestible.

Seeds and nuts can be used in various ways in food preparation. They make a wonderful garnish on salads, vegetable dishes, and casseroles. You can also eat them as a main source of protein with snacks and light meals. Many natural food stores and some supermarkets carry a variety of delicious seed and nut butters. Almond butter and sesame butter, which are high in calcium, are particularly good spreads. Both are delicious and are wonderful sources of nutrients. They are also very filling, so a little bit goes a long way. I recommend buying the raw nut and seed butters rather than the roasted ones.

Heating seeds and nuts is not desirable, since this process alters the integrity of their fatty acids. Nuts and seeds can also be made into flour, milk, and a variety of other food products.

Nut and seed oils can be used in salad dressings, sauces, sautés, and baked goods. They should not, however, be used in frying or be heated to high temperatures. Heat can alter their chemical structure and adversely affect the body's ability to process them. In fact, when cooking, it is best to use the more stable monounsaturated oils like olive or canola oils.

When choosing these oils, be sure to read labels carefully. The best quality oils are labeled "cold pressed." This type of processing helps to retain the fat-soluble vitamins A and D present in the oils. Heated or chemically extracted oils are less desirable to use in food preparation since the oils are altered in processing.

Recommended seed and nut oils include sesame oil, sunflower oil, almond oil, and walnut oil, to name a few. Of special note for food preparation is flax seed oil. This oil is one of my personal favorites. It has a rich, golden color and is an excellent butter substitute to sprinkle on vegetables, rice, potatoes, pasta, and popcorn. Unlike butter, flax oil cannot be used for cooking. Cook the foods first and add flax oil for flavoring just before serving. Pumpkin seed oil is also delicious, with its deep green color and spicy flavor. It is probably more difficult to find than flax seed oil.

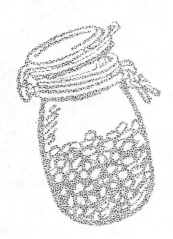

BEST SEEDS AND NUTS FOR DIETARY USE

Seeds	**Nuts**
Flax	Almond
Pumpkin	Filberts
Sesame	Pecans
Sunflower	Pistachios
	Walnuts

Fish and Poultry

Fish and poultry are the best choices for women who feel that they need to retain meat in their diet. A number of people simply enjoy the flavor and texture of meat, while a minority actually don't feel as well or as energized on an all-vegetarian diet.

If you fall into one of these categories, fish and poultry can supply a number of important nutritional needs. Both are excellent sources of high-quality protein. All types of fish, including saltwater fish, freshwater fish, and shellfish, as well as all types of commonly-eaten poultry like chicken, turkey, duck, goose, and game fowl, contain a complete range of the essential amino acids needed to build protein. These acids can be utilized by the body for many purposes, such as building structural components of tissue and maintaining immune function.

Many fish are also excellent sources of polyunsaturated fats, which provide tremendous health benefits. The best fish sources of these fats include salmon, trout, mackerel, and halibut.

Fish oils, including eicosapentanoic acid (EPA) and docosahexanoic acid (DHA), are converted to the series-3 prostaglandin hormones. One member of the series, called PGE 3, has anticlotting effects and helps to reduce platelet stickiness. As a result, it helps reduce the likelihood of heart attacks and strokes when it is manufactured by the body in high levels. PGE 3 also helps to decrease triglyceride levels, thereby reducing another risk factor for heart attacks. It also helps prevent the manufacture of PGE 2, an undesirable prostaglandin made from arachidonic acid, which is a fatty acid derived primarily from dietary sources of red meat and dairy products. Unlike PGE 3, arachidonic acid-derived PGE 2 actually promotes platelet aggregation or clumping, thereby initiating potentially dangerous clot formation.

The fats found in poultry are a different story. While poultry such as turkey, chicken, and goose do contain some of the beneficial linoleic acid, the amount is much less than that found in plant sources. Linoleic acid ranges between 15 to 20 percent of the total fat content of turkey and chicken and 20 to 25 percent in goose. Certain fish (like salmon and trout) are far better sources of essential fatty acids than poultry. Luckily, much of poultry's fat is found within the skin (which is laden with fat) and in the internal organs, so it can be easily removed. In addition, the total fat content of the most commonly eaten poultry—chicken, and turkey—is far lower than that of beef (11 percent for chicken, compared to 30 to 40 percent for beef).

If you want to minimize your fat intake when eating poultry, choose muscle meat like breast and thigh over the internal organs, and remove the skin before cooking or eating. Also, it is best to eat white meat rather than dark, as white meat is much lower in fat. Also, avoid duck and goose, which tend to contain more fat in their meat and skins.

Besides protein and fat, fish and poultry contain a number of other important nutrients. Fatty fish, such as salmon and halibut, are good sources of vitamins A and D. Mackerel, herring, and haddock tend to be rich in minerals, although this varies by type of fish. Saltwater fish and shellfish are excellent sources of iodine, a difficult-to-obtain trace mineral needed for healthy thyroid function. They are also high in zinc—particularly oysters, though lobster and crab are fairly abundant in zinc as well. Shellfish are also a good source of selenium and copper. In general, fish provide high quantities of potassium, phosphorus, and iron, though magnesium levels tend to be low. Fish can be an excellent source of calcium. Canned sardines and salmon are good choices because of their tiny, partially dissolved and easily digested bones.

Chicken and turkey are less abundant in their vitamin and mineral content, for the most part, than fish or vegetable sources. Chicken does contain some vitamin A and vitamin B complex, but no vitamin E and negligible amounts of vitamin C. It does contain some potassium, phosphorus, sodium, zinc, and iron, but levels of other minerals like calcium, magnesium, and manganese tend to be low.

Turkey is fairly similar to chicken in its nutrient makeup. A few minerals, such as potassium and phosphorus, are slightly more abundant in turkey than in chicken, but turkey's vitamin A content is even lower. Neither type of poultry should be used to supply all your vitamin and mineral needs. They should be combined with plant-based foods such as fruit, vegetables, and whole grains, which are richer in these essential micronutrients. The same is true, to a lesser extent, with seafood.

Seafood and poultry can be purchased fresh, frozen, canned, and smoked. Seafood is also available cured and dried. Both seafood and poultry are prone to bacterial contamination and can cause infections to the consumer if not handled properly. Neither type of meat should be left out at room temperature. They should be well wrapped, refrigerated, and eaten soon after purchasing or thawing.

Both fish and poultry are best eaten broiled, roasted, sautéed, or baked. Frying or sautéing in large amounts of fat should be avoided. Poultry is rarely eaten raw, although seafood in sushi bars and in some seafood recipes calls for it to be served raw or only lightly cooked. There is some risk of contamination by parasites and bacteria when eating raw or undercooked seafood. It is important that any seafood eaten this way be as fresh and clean as possible.

If you eat poultry frequently, try to buy the organic, range-fed brands, as their exposure to pesticides, antibiotics, and hormones has been reduced. Also, I recommend limiting your intake of meat to small portions (3 ounces or less per day). Most Americans eat much more protein than is healthy. Excessive amounts of protein are difficult to digest and stress the kidneys. Instead of using meat as your only source of protein, increase your intake of grains, beans, raw seeds, and nuts, which contain not only protein but also many other important nutrients. For many years I have recommended that my patients use meat more as a garnish and a flavoring for casseroles, stir-fries, and soups.

Types of Poultry

Chicken	Goose
Duck	Guinea hen
Game bird: pheasant, partridge, quail	Turkey

Types of Seafood

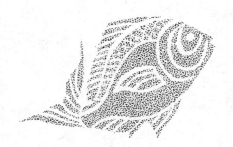

Freshwater Fish: trout, perch, pike, whitefish, catfish, bass, blue gill, crappie, crayfish, carp

Saltwater Fish: salmon, tuna, swordfish, shark, mackerel, sole, blue fish, flounder, red snapper, sardine, herring, smelt

Shellfish: crab, lobster, shrimp, scallop, abalone, oyster, mussel, clam

Fruits

Fruits are the edible structure of flowering plants, specifically the mature ovary of the plant. (This is why when we open up a fruit we see their seeds or the offspring of the plants.) Fruits come in many shapes and colors. They delight our senses with their sweet flavors and delicious textures. Nutritionally, fruits are a treasure trove of vitamins A and C, many minerals, natural sugars, fiber, and water. Some fruits even contain protein and fat. Many studies have been done on the abundant nutrients found in fruit. Adequate fruit intake can help to prevent or relieve a wide variety of female-related health complaints, as well as many general health problems. Fruits are an excellent source of vitamin C, which provides important protection against cancer and heart disease. In fact, vitamin C helps protect the cardiovascular system by preventing oxidation of the low-density lipoprotein cholesterol (LDL cholesterol). This is an early event leading to the development of atherosclerosis. Certain cancers, such as cervical cancer, occur more frequently in vitamin C-deficient individuals. Vitamin C reduces capillary fragility and can help control or reduce heavy menstrual flow in susceptible women, particularly in teenage girls and in women who are transitioning into menopause.

Vitamin C also has important antistress and immune stimulant properties. It is needed by the adrenals for the production of adrenal cortical hormones. Women who are deficient in vitamin C due to low dietary intake or insufficient supplementation tend to handle stress less effectively, resulting in anxiety, nervous tension, and even chronic fatigue. Adequate vitamin C intake helps us to fight off a wide range of viral and bacterial infections. Vitamin C is also needed for collagen production, which maintains the structural integrity of the skin. The best fruit sources of vitamin C include citrus fruits like oranges, grapefruits, tangerines, and lemons, and other fruits such as melons, strawberries, and other berries.

Citrus fruits and berries are also rich in bioflavonoids, another essential nutrient that affects blood vessel strength and permeability. Bioflavonoids also have an anti-inflammatory effect, important to women with allergies, menstrual cramps, or arthritis. Many bioflavonoids are natural sources of plant estrogens. Like our own endogenous estrogen, these weak dietary sources of estrogen can be supportive of the female reproductive tract and can improve mood and increase energy levels in women with PMS or menopausal symptoms. They can also help relieve estrogen-related migraine headaches. Although citrus fruits are excellent sources of bioflavonoids and vitamin C, they are highly acidic and may be difficult to digest for some women with food allergies or sensitive digestive tracts.

Citrus fruits are used for the commercial production of bioflavonoid supplements. Unfortunately, much of the bioflavonoids in citrus fruits are found in the inner peel and pulp of the fruit. This is the bitter part of the fruit that many people discard, unaware of its health benefits. Also, the skin of grapes, cherries, and many berries are rich sources of bioflavonoids. Make sure to eat the whole fruit rather than just the juice.

Yellow and orange fruits such as cantaloupe, papaya, persimmons, apricots, and tangerines should be included in your diet because of their high vitamin A content. Vitamin A in fruits is available in high levels as a provitamin called beta carotene. Like vitamin C, vitamin A helps to protect the body from developing many types of cancer, including cervical, lung, and bladder cancer. It also helps to protect the cardiovascular system from heart attacks and lowers the risk of strokes.

Vitamin A in the form of beta carotene helps to improve female health in a number of other ways. Deficiencies in vitamin A have been linked to benign breast disease, heavy menstrual bleeding, and skin aging. Because it is needed for healthy mucous membranes, a lack of vitamin A can worsen the signs of aging of the vagina and genitourinary tract after menopause. Vitamin A is also essential for healthy immune function, resistance to infection, and healthy vision. Clearly, beta carotene-containing fruit should be eaten often for adequate intake of this essential nutrient.

All fruits are excellent sources of potassium, though bananas, grapefruits, berries, peaches, apricots, raisins, figs, and melons are particularly rich in this important mineral. Adequate potassium intake is necessary for good health. It helps to regulate fluid balance in the body. When women are deficient in potassium at the expense of high levels of sodium (which is ubiquitous in the American diet as table salt), health problems can occur. Low potassium and high sodium levels can predispose a person to bloating and fluid retention during the premenstrual period. In women entering menopause, a potassium deficiency can worsen fluid retention, weight gain, and high blood pressure. Women with a low potassium intake tend to tire easily and lack stamina and endurance. In fact, several studies have shown that energy levels improve significantly when a combination of potassium and magnesium supplements are taken.

Besides containing high levels of potassium, certain fruits—raisins, blackberries, and bananas, to name a few—are good sources of calcium and magnesium. You can eat these fruits often, as their minerals are essential for proper nervous system and muscular function.

Eat fruits whole to benefit from their fiber, which helps to prevent constipation and other digestive irregularities.

Fresh and dried fruits are excellent snacks and dessert substitutes for cookies, candies, cakes, and other foods high in refined sugar. Although fruit is high in sugar, its fiber helps slow down absorption of the sugar into the blood and, thereby, helps stabilize the blood sugar level. Fruit juice, however, is another story, and I recommend consuming it in small quantities. While fruit juice contains nutrients like vitamin C and minerals, it does not contain the bulk or fiber of the whole fruit. As a result, it acts more like table sugar and can destabilize your blood sugar level dramatically when taken excessively. It can worsen anxiety, mood swings, fatigue, and "spaciness" in women with both hypoglycemia and PMS. In the case of fruit juice, less is better. If you want to have fruit juice on a more frequent basis, mix it with one-half water. It is best to drink it freshly squeezed right from the fruit since its nutrient content will be higher. If you cannot drink fruit juice right away, don't let it sit on the kitchen counter. Be sure to refrigerate it right away to protect its vitamin C.

A wide variety of fruits are available year-round, particularly apples, bananas, oranges, and grapefruits. These staples of the American diet are great breakfast foods. Enjoy seasonal fruits such as apricots, peaches, berries, cherries, melons, and the other delicious fruits that are available only briefly during the year. Try to eat locally grown fruits in season, as they will tend to be riper and fresher. Be sure to wash all fresh fruits before eating them. This will ensure that any chemical residue (or contamination) is removed. Eat the fruits whole or thinly peeled so that the nutrients found in the skin are preserved. Also, try to find unsprayed and organic fruit, if possible, to avoid pesticide exposure. Many supermarkets are beginning to carry unsprayed foods because of the strong consumer demand for clean products.

Besides fresh fruits, many varieties of frozen, canned, and dried fruits are available in supermarkets and grocery stores. Frozen fruits, if properly processed, may be similar in nutrient content to fresh fruits. However, loss of nutrients does occur in the canning and drying process. If you choose to buy canned fruits, be sure to avoid those in heavy, sugary syrup. Instead, buy canned fruit packed in its own juice or water.

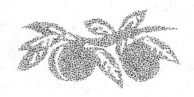

TYPES OF FRUITS

Temperate Climate Fruits
Apples
Pears
Plums

Citrus Fruits
Grapefruit
Lemons
Limes
Oranges
Tangelos
Tangerines

Cherries
Bing
Queen Anne

Melons
Cantaloupe
Casabas
Persian honeydews
Watermelons

Berries
Blackberries
Blueberries
Boysenberries
Cranberries
Gooseberries
Lingonberries
Raspberries
Strawberries

Grapes
Red seedless
Reiber
Thompson seedless

Tropical and Subtropical Fruits
Avocados
Bananas
Guavas
Kiwis
Papayas
Pineapples

Olives
Black olives
Green olives

Vegetables

The term "vegetables" refers to any herbaceous plant that can be eaten whole or in part. This can include the tubers, roots, stems, leaves, seeds, and flowering parts of the plant. These excellent foods come in a multitude of flavors, colors, and textures. They are composed primarily of water and carbohydrates and contain little protein or fat. They are also rich sources of many essential vitamins and minerals and provide needed bulk and fiber to the diet.

In the past few decades, many studies have concluded that the nutrients found in vegetables play an important role in protecting us from health problems. These essential nutrients include vitamin A, vitamin C, calcium, magnesium, potassium, iron, iodine, and more. In addition, vegetables contain other chemicals that help protect against heart attacks and boost immune function. Starchy vegetables help regulate blood sugar levels.

The form of vitamin A found in foods is beta carotene, a provitamin which is converted to vitamin A once it's taken into the body through the diet by the liver and intestines. Beta carotene is found in high doses in fruits and vegetables and is quite safe. For example, one glass of carrot juice or a sweet potato each contain 20,000 IU of beta carotene. Many people eat two to three times this amount in their daily diet. In contrast, high doses of supplemental vitamin A derived from fish liver oil can accumulate in the liver to toxic levels.

Vegetables high in vitamin A tend to have an orange, red, or dark green color. These include squash, sweet potatoes, yams, peppers, carrots, kale, spinach, turnip greens, collards, green onions, and romaine lettuce, among others. You should eat these foods often because research demonstrates that vitamin A can protect against cancer and immune problems. In women who are prone to allergies and infections, sufficient vitamin A intake can help bolster immune protection by strengthening the cell walls and mucous membranes. This protects against developing respiratory disease, as well as allergic episodes. In addition, research has linked low vitamin A levels to breast cancer, cervical cancer, bladder cancer, prostate cancer, lung cancer, and benign breast disease.

Vitamin A can play an important role in maintaining the health of women during their menopausal transition and postmenopausal years. One study from the University of South Africa found that women with heavy menstrual bleeding (a common problem as women transition into menopause) had lower blood vitamin A levels than normal volunteers.

Other studies suggest that a high intake of beta carotene-containing foods protects against heart attacks in high-risk people. The *Nurse's Health Study*, sponsored by Harvard University Medical School found that women consuming 15 to 20 mg per day of beta carotene had a 40 percent lower risk of strokes and a 22 percent lower risk of heart attacks when compared to women consuming less than 6 mg per day. Vitamin A deficiency has also been linked to fatigue, night blindness, skin aging, loss of smell, loss of appetite, and softening of bones and teeth.

Many vegetables are high in vitamin C. These include brussels sprouts, broccoli, cauliflower, kale, peppers, parsley, peas, tomatoes, and potatoes. Vitamin C helps to strengthen capillaries and prevent capillary fragility, thereby facilitating the flow of essential nutrients throughout the body and the excretion of waste products out of the body. This is particularly important for women transitioning into menopause who are prone to heavy menstrual bleeding. When used in combination with bioflavonoid-containing foods like soy, alfalfa, and buckwheat, foods high in vitamin C can actually help decrease menstrual flow. Vitamin C is also an important antistress vitamin because it is needed for healthy adrenal hormone production (the adrenal glands help us deal with stress). This is particularly important for women with anxiety due to emotional causes, allergies, or stress from other origins. Vitamin C is also important for immune function and wound healing. Its anti-infectious properties may help to reduce the tendency toward respiratory, bladder, and vaginal infections. Research also suggests that along with vitamin A, vitamin C may help protect women from developing cervical cancer.

Vegetables are also outstanding foods for their high mineral content. Many vegetables are high in calcium, magnesium, and potassium, which help to relieve and prevent the symptoms of menstrual cramps and PMS. Besides helping to relax tense muscles, these minerals also calm the emotions. Both calcium and magnesium act as natural tranquilizers, a benefit for women suffering from menstrual pain, discomfort, and irritability. Potassium aids in relieving the symptoms of premenstrual bloating by reducing fluid retention. Some of the best sources for these minerals include Swiss chard, spinach, broccoli, beet greens, mustard greens, sweet potatoes, kale, potatoes, peas, and green beans. These vegetables are also high in iron, which may also help to reduce cramps. In addition, the calcium, magnesium, potassium, and iron found in vegetables also help protect against the development of anemia, osteoporosis, and excessive menstrual bleeding.

These minerals can also increase and maintain energy levels. Calcium, magnesium, and potassium help to improve stamina, endurance, and vitality. Clinical studies have shown that supplemental magnesium and potassium reduce depression and increase energy levels dramatically. Iodine and trace minerals are essential for healthy thyroid function and thus, maintaining a steady energy level; vegetables like kelp and other types of seaweed are high in these minerals.

Vegetables contain not only high levels of vitamins and minerals, but also other chemicals that help prevent heart attacks and boost immune function. Onions and garlic decrease blood clotting and lower serum cholesterol, which can decrease the incidence of stroke and heart attack. Garlic has also been found to prevent and slow tumor growths in animals. Studies indicate that ginger root, onions, and mushrooms may have a similar effect. Certain mushrooms may even stimulate immune function. Vegetables like broccoli and cauliflower contain chemicals called indoles and isothiocyanates, which help block the activation of carcinogens, such as tobacco smoke, before they cause harm the body.

Potatoes, sweet potatoes, and yams are starches—soft, well-tolerated carbohydrates. Like other complex carbohydrates, starches calm the mood by helping to regulate the blood sugar level. You can steam, mash, and bake potatoes; eat them alone, or include them in other low-stress dishes and casseroles. Starches combine very well with a variety of vegetables and can form the basis of delicious, low-stress meals. Women deriving their dietary proteins primarily from vegetables sources can combine starches with lentils or split peas in soups or stews for a complete balance of amino acids.

In stores, you can buy fresh, raw vegetables, or vegetables that have been frozen, canned, or dried. Because raw vegetables are the freshest and contain the highest levels of vitamins and minerals, they are your best choice. However, quick-freezing techniques and proper canning do preserve nutrients quite well. Dried vegetables tend to exhibit the greatest loss of nutrients.

Eat as many raw vegetables as possible. You can enjoy a variety of raw vegetables in salads, or munch them with healthful dips. Fresh vegetable juice is another option. Though the fiber is discarded in the juicing process, the vitamins and minerals are retained. Juices can be quite easy to digest, but if you find that you do not tolerate raw vegetables well and they cause you digestive discomfort, cooking them may be preferable.

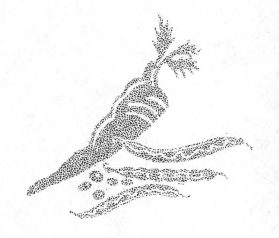

Cooking breaks down the fiber in the vegetables, making them softer and more digestible. Steaming is the best cooking method because it preserves essential nutrients. A woman with extreme stress and fatigue may even want to purée her steamed vegetables in a blender. However, as a woman begins to recover her energy level, she should add raw foods such as salads, juices, and raw vegetables to her meals for more texture and variety. Do not boil vegetables; vitamins and minerals can be lost by overcooking them.

Before eating fresh vegetables, be sure to wash them thoroughly to remove any pesticides, herbicides, and dirt. Some women even wash their vegetables in a dilute solution of bleach (Clorox) if they are concerned about chemical contamination. Leave the skin of the vegetable intact or pare it thinly because many nutrients are concentrated in this part of the plant. And be sure to store fresh vegetables in the refrigerator soon after obtaining them to avoid loss of nutrients.

VEGETABLE GROUPS

Gourds
Acorn squash
Butternut squash
Chayote
Crook-neck
Squash
Cucumber
Pumpkin
Zucchini squash

Cruciferous Vegetables
Broccoli
Brussels sprouts
Cabbage
Cauliflower

Root Vegetables
Beets
Carrots
Garlic
Onions
Radishes
Rutabagas
Turnips

Nightshades
Chili pepper
Eggplant
Garden pepper
Paprika
Potatoes
Sweet potatoes
Tomatoes

Leafy Greens
Chard
Kale
Lettuce
Spinach

Mushrooms
Button
Shiitake

Sweeteners

The purpose of sweeteners is to provide concentrated flavor to a variety of beverages, baked goods, desserts, and other food products. Sweeteners also provide a rapidly absorbed source of energy to the body since they are usually simple sugars. Unfortunately, sweeteners (particularly table sugar made from beets or sugar cane) are overused in our society. When used to excess, they can destabilize the blood sugar level, promote obesity and the overgrowth of candida, adversely affect mood and energy levels, and promote tooth decay. In small amounts, however, sweeteners can impart a delicious flavor to foods.

The best quality (and most delicious) sweeteners include honey, maple syrup, rice bran syrup, fruit juice, molasses, and carob. With the exception of molasses and carob, most sweeteners are not high in nutrients. Molasses, the residue from the processing of beet or cane sugar, is a thick, syrupy liquid that is brown in color and has a strong flavor. Unlike table sugar, molasses is rich in nutrients. It is an excellent source of calcium (one tablespoon contains 137 mg of calcium), magnesium, iron, copper, and other minerals. Molasses is also rich in vitamins B and E. As a sweetener, molasses imparts its delicious, distinct flavor to baked goods, and combines well with spices like cinnamon, ginger, and allspice. Carob is a natural sweetener with a flavor and appearance similar to chocolate. In fact, carob is often used as a chocolate or cocoa substitute because it is caffeine-free (chocolate and cocoa contain a fair amount of caffeine). Carob is a fairly good source of protein, calcium, and phosphorus. It is a versatile flavoring, available in powder, syrup, and block forms for different uses.

While honey does not have the nutrient benefits of molasses and carob, it stands out as a sweetener. It is a flower extract digested and regurgitated by bees who store it in their hives. Honey has a beautiful texture and color which can vary depending on the flower and site from which the honey is gathered. It is twice as sweet as table sugar, so you can use it in smaller amounts. This factor alone would make it preferable to table sugar for food preparation. Honey is often used in baked goods and other sweetened products available in natural food stores.

Maple syrup is a delicious, light brown liquid sweetener obtained by tapping the sap from maple trees. It is commonly used on breakfast foods like pancakes and waffles. Manufacturers of natural food products increasingly use it much like honey to sweeten cereals and baked goods. When choosing maple syrup, it is important to read the label on the can or bottle carefully to make sure that it is genuine. There are imitation maple syrup products on the market. They look like maple syrup, but are really just corn syrup with a small bit of maple syrup added to justify the label claim. If it is the genuine product, maple syrup should be the only ingredient listed on the label. Also, Canadian manufacturing practices are better than those in the United States, so buy Canadian syrup if you can. In this country, manufacturers are allowed to use formaldehyde on their trees to improve sap production. Formaldehyde is a toxic chemical which contaminates any food and should be avoided.

Fruit juice is another sweetener that can be used when preparing baked goods like cakes, frozen desserts, marinades, sauces, and other types of foods. Apple and grape juice are used to sweeten commercially prepared food products. They impart the distinctive flavor of the whole fruit, a delicious benefit. Fruit juices contain fructose, the same type of sugar found in honey. Fructose is twice as sweet as sucrose, the sweetener found in sugar. Be careful, as drinking fruit juice in large quantities can destabilize the blood sugar level and worsen the symptoms of hypoglycemia and PMS.

Finally, stevia is an herbal-based sweetener. It can be used as a sweetener by women with hypoglycemia or diabetes. Since it contains no calcium from sugar (only imparting the flavor of sweeteners), it does not imbalance the blood sugar level. Unfortunately, at the present time, the U.S. Food and Drug Administration (FDA) has disallowed its commercial sale.

Sweeteners (Other than Table Sugar)

Carob	Molasses
Maple syrup	Stevia

Herbs and Spices

Seasonings are used to impart a variety of flavors to food and can greatly enhance the enjoyment of our meals. Seasonings come from plant sources and are derived from many different parts of the plant itself. Common herbs originate from the root of plants (ginger, licorice), leaves (basil, dill, tarragon, oregano), seeds (mustard, poppy, celery), and berries (black pepper, cayenne). While many of these spices do have some nutritive content, they are usually used in quantities too small to affect our nutrient status. For example, one teaspoon of cumin contains 1.4 mg of iron, but only tiny amounts of calcium and magnesium. Celery seed is a slightly better source of calcium, with one teaspoon containing 35 mg of calcium and 0.9 mg of iron. On the whole, spices should be used to make foods more flavorful and attractive rather than as significant sources of vitamins and minerals.

Herbal seasonings and spices tend to lose their potency fairly rapidly. In fact, the more aromatic they are, the more readily this occurs. To preserve their flavoring and scent, all spices should be stored in tightly covered jars and containers, away from sunlight. Unused spices sitting on the shelf should be replaced after six months since their potency tends to fade after this period of time. Bulk herbs available in natural food stores tend to be much less expensive than prebottled herbs in supermarkets.

Herbs and spices are also available as liquid extracts. These products capture the flavor of plants such as vanilla bean, peppermint, lemon, and almond and are sold in alcohol or water mixtures. Thus, the essence of the plant is concentrated with little nutrient value. Extracts can be very useful as flavoring agents for baked goods, frozen desserts, candies, and beverages. Like the plants themselves, extracts should be kept out of sunlight and stored in dark glass bottles to prevent rapid aging of the product.

PLANT SOURCES OF HERBS AND SPICES

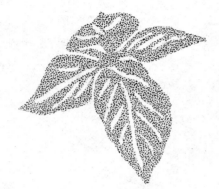

Leaves	Roots	Seeds
Basil	Ginger	Celery
Dill	Licorice	Mustard
Oregano		Poppy
Tarragon	**Berries**	
	Black pepper	
	Cayenne	

Water

Water is essential to life since it comprises 60 to 70 percent of our bodies (the percentage is higher in infants than in older people). Not only do humans depend on water to survive and flourish, but so do all animals and plants on the earth.

Water is the main liquid that we drink, cook with, and clean our foods with. Though we can live for a period of time without food, this is not so with water. We must take in water on a daily basis to survive in optimal health (or to survive at all).

Since we lose water constantly through our skin, lungs, urinary tract, and bowels, sufficient replacement of it through our foods and beverages is mandatory. About half our water needs can be met through food intake. Particularly good sources are water-rich foods like fruits and vegetables. Denser foods like meat, seeds, and nuts do not provide as much water for our daily needs. Most people find that they also need to drink 6 to

8 glasses per day of water to maintain their fluid balance adequately. During very hot weather, we may need to drink even more to avoid the effects of fluid loss and dehydration. This need also increases during times of physical stress such as illness when there is increased fluid loss due to fever or diarrhea.

The quality of our water is very important. We depend on it for our health and well-being. Much of the fresh water on the earth has been contaminated by chemical pollutants, fertilizers, industrial wastes, air pollutants, and animal wastes. As a result, many of us question how safe the water really is coming out of our taps, with good reason.

Analysis of various municipal and artesian well water has found significant levels of pollutants like lead, mercury, organic solvents, and nitrates which are not removed by our current water treatment practices. The quality of water is made even worse by the widespread use of chlorine, an anti-infective agent used to destroy pathogens like bacteria, but which itself breaks down into a variety of carcinogenic chemicals. Many safer alternative water treatments, like purification with an ozone-oxygen mixture, are used extensively in the municipal water systems of European countries and other countries, but have not come into widespread use in the United States.

What can you do to ensure an excellent quality of drinking water? There are currently four options available: installing home filtration, using purification systems, buying spring water or distilled water from a commercial source, or using a well on your own property.

• **Home filtration systems** are probably the best and least expensive way to ensure good quality water for your personal needs. Apparently many Americans agree, as they are buying several million of these units a year. While units differ in their type of filtration and purification systems, good quality systems will remove or destroy almost all of the bacteria, heavy metals, and chemicals that remain in the water.

- The most commonly used **purification systems** employ one of the following:
    1. carbon filters, which attract and absorb pollutants.
    2. reverse osmosis, which passes the water through several different micropore membranes that trap the pollutants.
    3. distillation, which consists of vaporizing water or turning it into steam in one chamber and condensing it back into liquid in a second chamber, removing pollutants in the process.
    4. ozone-oxygen purification systems, which effectively kill all bacteria, viruses, and other pathogens; cause heavy metals to flocculate or clump together so that they can be effectively filtered out; and oxidize chemical pollutants to harmless by-products. The best purification systems do not use a single method but instead employ a combination of these techniques to ensure the most complete removal of toxins and pollutants.
- You can purchase **spring water,** which is available from many bottling companies throughout the United States. Spring water comes from underground springs or fresh surface water reservoirs. Other than being treated to kill bacteria and other pathogens, often by chlorine, this water is not processed. Many people feel that spring water has a better flavor than tap water and buy it specifically for this reason. If you are concerned about the issue of contaminants in the spring water you buy, it is a good idea to ask the company for a summary of laboratory tests on water quality. A company with high standards will have their water quality checked at least annually by an independent laboratory.
- In several areas, water can come from **a well** on the property rather than a municipal water system. This type of water

can vary greatly in quality. Some well water is quite "soft," lacking many minerals while others are "hard" and rich in minerals such as calcium, magnesium, iron, selenium, and other beneficial nutrients. The major concern with well water is potential contamination by pesticides, herbicides, asbestos, toxic heavy metals, bacterial pathogens, and other pollutants. If you depend on a well for your water needs, be sure to have it analyzed for these pollutants. If it checks out in all areas of safety, well water can be an excellent source of fresh water. If there are areas of concern, be sure to purchase a good home filtration system if you wish to continue using a well as your main source of water.

CHAPTER 2

Foods to Avoid or Limit

*T*his chapter deals with the health risks that many commonly eaten foods in our society pose for women (and men also). The list of hazardous foods may surprise you because it includes not only processed "junk food," but also foods that are considered staples of the American diet. Many women unwittingly prescribe to a diet that worsens their reproductive health as well as their health in general.

The wrong foods can affect health adversely in many ways. They can be difficult to digest, contain nutrients that stress the body, or even cause toxic reactions within the body.

The process of digestion itself takes much energy. Digestion must occur before the body can extract energy from the foods you eat. Proteins must be broken down into amino acids, complex carbohydrates into simple sugars, and fats into fatty acids. For these breakdowns to occur, food is chemically acted upon by stomach acid, hormones, pancreatic enzymes, and fat emulsifiers, as well as by the mechanical process that propels food through the entire length of the digestive tract. Once the food is broken down, it must be absorbed from the digestive tract and taken into the blood. From there, the food particles circulate to cells throughout the body. At the cellular level, the energy contained in the food is finally captured to fuel the body's many chemical and physiological reactions.

This entire process requires a great deal of work. The body needs an abundance of reserve energy to produce the chemicals involved in the digestive process. Ideally, foods should be easy to digest, yet nutrient-rich, so that they can provide the body with needed energy.

Unfortunately, many of the most commonly eaten foods in our society are hard to digest. These include foods that are high in saturated fats, sugars, and animal protein. The long list includes pizza, steak, bacon, cheeseburgers, hot dogs, French fries, doughnuts, ice cream, chocolate, and many other processed and high-stress foods. The body must work very hard to digest a typical meal of thick steak, French fries, buttered bread, wine, and a chocolate dessert. This meal is laden with saturated fats, red meat protein, and sugar. Upon finishing it, a woman will feel overly full and more tired than before she started eating. In contrast, a light meal of bean soup, mixed green salad, and baked potato is filled with vitamins, minerals, carbohydrates, and easy-to-digest vegetable-based protein. This meal is also low in fat and sugar. It is much more likely to enable that woman to leave the table feeling energized and comfortable.

Other foods stress the body through their toxicity. There are many ways a food can increase fatigue. Some foods have a toxic effect that damages the cells and affects their ability to function. One example is alcohol, which is particularly toxic to the liver, brain, and nervous system. Alcohol and sugar promote the growth of pathological organisms like candida, which can worsen fatigue. Many food additives and preservatives can cause an allergic or toxic reaction in susceptible women. Other foods, such as saturated fats, margarine, caffeine, salt, and food additives, will be discussed in the following sections of this chapter for their adverse affects on health.

Caffeine

Caffeine-containing foods include coffee, black tea, cola drinks, cocoa, and chocolate. These foods are used almost universally in our culture both as stimulants and emotional "treats." Caffeine belongs to a class of chemicals called methylxanthines, which have a druglike stimulant effect on the body. In fact, caffeine-containing foods are the most commonly used legal drugs (along with alcohol) in Western societies. For thousands of years, people have used caffeine in rituals and ceremonies. It was also chewed in plant form or used in beverages as a mild daily stimulant. Traditional societies today continue to use caffeine-containing plants like mate or kola nuts for their stimulatory effects.

In the United States, many of us are unknowingly raised on caffeine-containing foods from our childhood. Hot chocolate is a favorite drink of children, especially during the winter months. Teenagers drink copious amounts of colas and other caffeine-containing carbonated drinks, and most children name chocolate as their preferred sweet. Among adults, coffee use is ubiquitous, with Americans consuming as much as ten pounds of coffee per year. Even more staggering is the statistic that Americans consume a half billion cups of coffee per day (or about two cups per person each day). These figures have decreased by 50 percent over the past forty years when coffee consumption was at its peak. A single cup of coffee contains about 100 mg of caffeine, enough to create a mild stimulatory effect.

Black tea and green tea contain about half the amount of caffeine that coffee does (about 50 mg per cup). However, these teas also contain theophylline and theobromine, other members of the methylxanthine family which have marked effects on the body. Theophylline is used as a medication to aid breathing in asthmatics, while theobromine has stimulatory effects on the body. Both tea and coffee contain tannic acid, which can irritate the intestinal mucosa. Theobromine is also found in the cocoa bean, the natural source of chocolate and cocoa powder used in cooking. Other plant sources of caffeine include mate, kola nuts, and the guarana plant.

Many soft drinks like Pepsi-Cola, Coca-Cola, Dr. Pepper, and Jolt, are high in caffeine. Numerous over-the-counter medications also contain caffeine as an active ingredient. Manufacturers of cold remedies like Dristan use it for its stimulatory effect to help counteract the drowsiness caused by antihistamines. It is a main ingredient in over-the-counter drugs like No-Doz because of its ability to increase wakefulness and alertness. It is also used in many pain-relief and menstrual-relief formulas such as Midol, Excedrin, and Anacin.

As a central nervous system stimulant, caffeine increases brain activity when taken in doses of 50 to 100 mg or more per day. This is the amount found in one cup of coffee or black tea. When used on an occasional basis, a cup of coffee can have a pleasantly stimulating effect. However, many people are addicted to the jolt of energy that caffeine provides and find that they need to take it in large amounts. Many women must consume significantly more caffeine (two to three cups or even as many as ten cups per day) to receive the pick-me-up they need to combat drowsiness and perform optimally during the day. Besides increasing alertness, caffeine has other physiological effects. It speeds up metabolism, allowing calories to be burned more efficiently. It stimulates the cardiovascular system, increasing the heart rate, respiratory rate, and elevating blood pressure. It lowers the blood sugar level, increasing the appetite and the craving for sweets. It also stimulates adrenal function, causing an outpouring of adrenal hormones which make the blood sugar level subsequently rise again. Caffeine also has a diuretic and laxative effect, increasing elimination.

Unfortunately, there are many negatives to the use of caffeinated beverages, which over time outweigh the initial benefits. Caffeine can cause a host of emotional and physical symptoms that can be quite debilitating. Caffeine is an addictive chemical, so many women find that they need increasingly larger amounts to keep their energy up. When caffeine use is initially discontinued, people tend to feel very fatigued. Women who suffer from PMS or menopause may find that psychological symptoms that can occur due to hormonal imbalance or deficiency—such as anxiety, irritability, and mood swings—are worsened with caffeine intake. In one study reported in the *American Journal of Public Health,* 216 female college students were questioned as to the severity of their PMS symptoms in relationship to their caffeine intake. Interestingly, only 16 percent of the women who used no caffeine at all reported suffering from severe PMS symptoms. In contrast, 60 percent of those women drinking between 4.5 to 15 cups of caffeinated beverages per day reported severe symptoms. This fourfold difference in frequency of symptoms is quite significant.

For women with anxiety and panic episodes due to emotional triggers, caffeine can aggravate the frequency and severity of their episodes. Caffeine taken in excess (more than four or five cups per day) can dramatically increase anxiety, irritability, and mood swings. Even small amounts can make susceptible women jittery. After the initial jolt, women with anxiety symptoms find that caffeine intake makes them more tired.

Caffeine triggers anxiety and panic symptoms because it directly stimulates arousal mechanisms in the body. It raises the brain's level of norepinephrine, a neurotransmitter that increases alertness. It also triggers sympathetic nervous system activity, which causes fight-or-flight responses, such as increased pulse, breathing rate, and muscle tension. Thus, caffeine intake triggers the physiological responses typical of anxiety states. In addition, caffeine stimulates the release of stress hormones from the adrenal glands, further intensifying nervousness and jitteriness. By overstimulating the adrenals, chronic use of caffeine actually weakens them. Over time, this can lead to persistent fatigue and tiredness.

Besides causing anxiety symptoms, caffeine has a diuretic effect and speeds elimination of many minerals and vitamins that are essential to health during the menopausal years. Loss of potassium, zinc, magnesium, vitamin B, and vitamin C are accelerated with caffeine intake. Many of these nutrients, such as B-complex vitamins and magnesium, are needed for optimal functioning of the chemical reactions that convert food to usable energy.

Deficiency of these nutrients increases anxiety, mood swings, and fatigue. Depletion of B-complex vitamins through caffeine use also interferes with carbohydrate metabolism and healthy liver function, which help to regulate the blood sugar as well as estrogen levels. An imbalance in estrogen and progesterone can increase anxiety and mood swings in women with symptoms of PMS or menopause. Many menopausal women also complain that caffeine increases the frequency of hot flashes.

Coffee also reduces the absorption of iron and calcium from food and supplemental sources, particularly when taken at mealtimes. This is obviously of concern to women who want to prevent osteoporosis and iron deficiency anemia.

Caffeine use has also been linked to a worsening of

nodularity and tenderness in women with benign breast disease. Studies published in both the *Journal of the American Medical Association* and *Surgery* reported decrease in breast pain as well as size of breast lumps for women when they eliminate caffeine from their diets. Many of my patients have reported a decrease in breast symptoms when discontinuing caffeine use. Women with frequent bladder infections or irritability and those suffering from interstitial cystitis, a debilitating chronic bladder disease, may also benefit from caffeine elimination.

Postmenopausal women who are at high risk of heart attacks and strokes due to their familial tendency or blood fat profiles may want to avoid caffeine use. Caffeine increases blood levels of cholesterol and triglycerides; both are risk factors for heart attacks. In addition, caffeine raises the blood pressure. High blood pressure, or hypertension, becomes increasingly prevalent with age and also is a risk factor for heart attacks and strokes. Caffeine also causes the heart beat faster and increases the excitability of the system that conducts electrical impulses through the heart. This can lead to rapid and irregular heartbeat in susceptible women.

Caffeine use directly affects hydrochloric acid secretion in the stomach. Specifically, caffeine increases acid production, which is a risk factor for gastritis and peptic ulcer disease. If you are prone to heartburn or either of these medical conditions, you should eliminate all caffeinated beverages for symptom relief. Besides triggering acid production, caffeine also stimulates peristalsis of the gastrointestinal tract. This has a laxative effect, producing more frequent bowel movements and even diarrhea in susceptible women. Too loose bowel movements can affect the loss of essential nutrients like B vitamins and minerals that are seen with the frequent use of caffeine.

Women who suffer from the side effects of caffeine or find

that it aggravates preexisting health conditions should cut down their caffeine intake substantially or eliminate it entirely from their diet. Habitual coffee, tea, cola, or cocoa drinkers should reduce their daily intake to one cup (or glass) per day or even less.

Unfortunately, women may find that going "cold turkey" with coffee and eliminating it abruptly causes unpleasant withdrawal symptoms such as headaches, depression, and fatigue. I have asked patients to abruptly stop caffeine usage on the weekends, when they were more relaxed and did not require the stimulation that caffeine provided. However, severe withdrawal headaches often ruined the leisure-time activities they planned on their days off.

To avoid uncomfortable withdrawal symptoms, it is better to cut down caffeine intake gradually. The best strategy is to decrease amounts slowly for one to several months. At the same time, other beverages can be substituted. Many of these substitutes either provide the taste or "look" of coffee. Certain beverages can even produce a similar pick-me-up without causing caffeine's deleterious effects. If you like the flavor of coffee, water process decaffeinated coffee is often the easiest substitute to start with. However, if you do use "decaf," be sure to buy a product prepared by steam distillation or the "Swiss water process" to remove the caffeine. Otherwise, you may be exposed to residues of dangerous chemicals like methyl chloride that are used in other methods of processing. Grain-based coffee substitutes, such as Pero, Postum, and Caffix, are even better. Ginger tea is a stimulant that can actually be therapeutic for women since it has a vitalizing and energetizing effect. Many of my patients make ginger tea by simply grating a few teaspoons of raw ginger root into a pot of water. It has a pleasant, spicy taste that many people enjoy. In addition, vitamins and mineral supplements and regular exercise can boost your energy levels without the use of coffee.

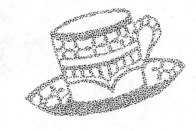

If you tend to be nervous and edgy in the morning, you might want to start the day with an herbal tea like chamomile or hops. These teas have a pleasant, relaxing, and calming effect.

CAFFEINE CONTENT OF BEVERAGES AND FOODS
(listed in order of caffeine content)

Product	Caffeine per Serving
Coffee	(per cup)
Drip (average)	146 mg
Percolated (average)	110 mg
Coffee (instant)	(per cup)
Folgers	97.5 mg
Maxwell House	94 mg
Nescafé	81
Decaffeinated Coffee	(per cup)
Sanka	4 mg
Brim	3.5 mg
Taster's Choice	3.5 mg
Tea	(per cup)
Tetley	63.5 mg
Lipton	52 mg
Constant Comment	29 mg
Soft Drinks	(per 12 oz. can)
Tab	56.6 mg
Mountain Dew	55 mg
Diet Dr. Pepper	54 mg
Coke Classic	46 mg
Diet Coke	46 mg
Pepsi	38.4 mg
Diet Pepsi	36 mg
Hot Chocolate Drinks	(per cup)
Cocoa	13 mg

Candy	(per oz.)
Ghirardelli Dark Chocolate	24 mg
Hershey's Milk Chocolate	4 mg

Side Effects of Caffeine Use

Anxiety, irritability, nervousness

Chronic fatigue

Depletion of potassium, magnesium, zinc, vitamin C, and vitamin B

Diarrhea

Dizziness

Frequent urination

Headaches

Heartburn

Insomnia, restlessness

Less absorption of iron and calcium

Rapid and irregular heartbeats

Conditions Worsened by the Use of Caffeine

Adrenal exhaustion

Anxiety

Chronic fatigue

Fibrocystic breast disease

Gastritis and ulcers

Hypertension

Insomnia

Interstitial cystitis

Menopausal symptoms

Osteoporosis

PMS

Alcohol

Alcoholic beverages are available in a wide variety of types and potencies. They are produced either by the fermentation of grains and fruits or the distillation of grains and starches. Alcohol has been taken for thousands of years, both as a social and commercial beverage. Today, there are over 100 million consumers of alcoholic beverages in the United States alone. Next to caffeine, alcohol is the most abused legal drug of choice for people wishing to alter their energy level and their mood.

Alcohol is a central nervous system depressant. Though it relaxes the drinker and has a mild tranquilizing effect, it also slows down physical processes. In addition, mental alertness and acuity are decreased when drinking alcohol. It is often difficult (if not impossible) for many people to perform demanding intellectual work after imbibing alcoholic beverages. Physical coordination and reflexes are also impaired when drinking, which is one reason why it is so dangerous to drive after drinking.

On the plus side, the relaxant effect of alcohol can remove inhibitions and improve congeniality at parties and other social gatherings. This is why people often socialize with a beer or a glass of wine in their hands. When consumed in small amounts, alcohol can promote a relaxed state of mind for people after a hard day of work, or enhance pleasure when they are socializing. An added benefit is that alcohol stimulates the appetite and increases the enjoyment of dining. There are even possible health benefits with moderate use. Alcohol improves blood circulation by dilating blood vessels and causes a mild increase in the beneficial HDL cholesterol, which is thought to decrease the risk of heart attacks.

Unfortunately, many people take alcohol in amounts far beyond that which is needed to produce the social or health benefits. In fact, 10 percent of all alcohol consumers in this country (10 million people) cannot limit their amount of alcohol use and are diagnosed as alcoholics. Many people abuse alcohol because they are trying to suppress strong emotions. Often, people increase their alcohol intake to unhealthy levels as an attempt to dull emotional pain and anxiety. It is also thought that alcoholics may have a genetic proclivity towards abuse, and it is true that alcoholism runs in families.

Some people may crave alcohol because they are allergic to the grains, grapes, or yeast from which the beverages are made. As with other food allergies, the sufferer may crave the food to which he or she is allergic. Thus, alcohol abuse in some people may be a manifestation of an underlying medical problem.

Alcohol, itself, has no particular nutritive value. It contains almost twice the calories of protein and carbohydrate foods (7 calories per gram versus 4 calories per gram, respectively). Unfortunately, these are empty calories. Alcohol is readily digested and easily absorbed from the digestive tract so it rapidly affects the blood sugar level after ingestion. Once absorbed, it is metabolized by the liver and used immediately as energy or stored as fat in the liver. Unfortunately, alcohol cannot be converted to storage forms of carbohydrate, which would be much more beneficial.

The excessive use of alcohol can significantly worsen a number of common female health problems, including PMS, menopausal symptoms, anxiety states, depression, heavy menstrual bleeding, fibroid tumors of the uterus, fibrocystic breast disease, and endometriosis.

Women with moderate to severe anxiety, mood swings, and depression due to PMS, menopause, or emotional causes, should avoid alcohol entirely or limit its use to occasional small amounts. Alcohol, like a simple sugar, is rapidly absorbed by the body. Like other sugars, alcohol increases hypoglycemia symptoms; excessive use can increase anxiety and mood swings. This can be particularly pronounced in women with PMS-related hypoglycemia.

As mentioned earlier, once alcohol has been absorbed and assimilated, it is metabolized primarily by the liver. This is a complex process requiring much work. Excessive intake of alcohol can overwhelm the liver's ability to process it, leading to toxic by-products that can themselves affect mood. Too much alcohol can also impede the body's ability to detoxify other chemicals—including drugs, hormones such as estrogen, and pesticides—that we take into our bodies by choice or through environmental contact. As a result, toxic levels of these chemicals can build up in the body, worsening anxiety.

The liver metabolizes estrogen, thus playing an important role in regulating estrogen levels in the body. Normally, the liver can metabolize estradiol, the main type of estrogen secreted by the ovaries, to less potent forms of estrogen as it passes through the hepatic circulation. When liver function is healthy, it will convert estradiol to estrone and estriol—the much weaker and less potent forms of estrogen. In the liver, estrogen is also inactivated by binding it to sulfates and gluccoronates. From there, the inactivated and weaker forms of estrogen are secreted into the bile and, finally, the intestinal tract. Much of the estrogen is then excreted from the body with the bowel movements.

When liver function is compromised by alcohol, estrogen levels can become elevated. This can be a risk factor for the aggravation of many common female problems such as heavy menstrual bleeding, fibroid tumors of the uterus, endometriosis, fibrocystic breast disease, and PMS.

During midlife and beyond, alcohol can actually intensify almost every type of menopause symptom. As a result, I recommend that women with active symptoms limit their intake or avoid alcoholic beverages entirely. The list of menopause symptoms affected by alcohol intake includes hot flashes and mood swings. Unlike caffeine, alcohol is a central nervous system depressant, so its intake can worsen menopausal fatigue and depression. This is particularly pronounced in women with night sweats and insomnia whose sleep quality is already poor. In addition, alcohol has a diuretic effect on the body. Estrogen helps keep the skin and other tissues plump by causing fluid and salt retention in the body. So, excessive intake of alcohol can further dehydrate the skin and tissues, including the vaginal and bladder mucosa, already at risk for dehydration because of estrogen deficiency. Alcohol's diuretic effect also causes the loss of excessive amounts of essential minerals through the urinary tract. These include minerals needed for healthy bones, such as calcium, magnesium, and zinc. Women who are addicted to alcohol may also have a negative calcium balance because of poor nutritional habits. Alcoholics often eat less calcium-rich food and ignore their intake of other essential nutrients, preferring the empty, nonnutritive calories of alcohol.

Alcohol, an irritant to the liver and other parts of the digestive tract, may be used by the body for immediate energy, or stored in the liver or in the rest of the body as fat. Unfortunately, the liver cannot convert alcohol to a storage form of glucose. As a result, the amount of fat stored in the liver increases with excessive alcohol use. Alcohol raises the liver enzyme level, leading to liver inflammation (or hepatitis). Eventually the chemical by-products of alcohol and the fat derived from alcohol can cause scarring and shrinkage of the liver, leading to its functional impairment and cirrhosis. In addition, alcohol irritates the lining of the upper digestive tract, including the esophagus, stomach, and upper part of the small intestine. It also causes irritation and inflammation of the pancreas. Over time, this can result in worsening of hypoglycemia and diabetes, as well as impaired absorption and assimilation of essential nutrients from the small intestine. Some of these nutrients, such as B vitamins, are necessary to stabilize these conditions.

The nervous system is particularly susceptible to the deleterious effects of alcohol, which readily crosses the blood-brain barrier and actually destroys brain cells. Alcohol can cause profound behavioral and psychological changes in women who drink it excessively. Symptoms include emotional upset, irrational anger, emotional outbursts, poor judgment, loss of memory, mental impairment, dizziness, poor coordination, and difficulty in walking.

Symptoms of emotional upset triggered by alcohol can also be due to candida overgrowth, since candida thrive on the sugar in alcohol. Alcohol can, thus, promote a tendency toward chronic candida infections. Women with candida-related mood upset and fatigue should avoid alcohol entirely. Furthermore, many women with allergies are sensitive to the yeast in alcohol, which worsens their allergic symptoms.

Fermented Alcoholic Beverages	Distilled Alcoholic Beverages
Ale	Rum
Beer	Rye
Port	Scotch
Sherry	Vodka
Stout	Whiskey
Wine	
Bourbon	
Gin	

PERCENT (%) ALCOHOL BY BEVERAGE

Beverage	Percent Alcohol
Beer	3 - 6
Bourbon	35 - 50
Gin	35 - 50
Port	12 - 18
Rum	35 - 50
Scotch	35 - 50
Sherry	12 - 18
Vodka	35 - 50
Whiskey	35 -50
Wine	9 - 12

When taken carefully—not exceeding 4 ounces of wine per day, 12 ounces of beer, or 1 ounce of hard liquor—alcohol can have a delightfully relaxing effect in women who are healthy. As mentioned earlier, it can make us more sociable and enhance the taste of food. For optimal health, however, I recommend drinking alcohol no more than once or twice a week. Women with preexisting health problems, particularly estrogen-related problems like PMS or fibroid tumors of the uterus, should avoid drinking alcohol entirely when they are symptomatic. Fortunately, there are many good alcohol substitutes. If you entertain a great deal and enjoy social drinking, try nonalcoholic beverages. A nonalcoholic cocktail, such as mineral water with a twist of lime, lemon, or a dash of bitters, is a good substitute. Near Beer is a nonalcoholic beer substitute that tastes almost like the real thing. Light wine and beer have a lower alcohol content than hard liquor, liqueurs, and regular wine. They can be mixed with mineral waters, crushed ice, or fresh fruit for a variety of delicious low-alcohol drinks.

Sugar and Artificial Sweeteners

Sugar is primarily used as a sweetening agent in the form of sucrose, which most of us know as white, granular "table sugar." It is one of the most overused foods in the Western world. Refined white sugar and brown sugar are the primary ingredients of cookies, cakes, soft drinks, candies, ice cream, cereals, and other sweet foods. In addition, foods such as pasta and bread—made out of white flour with the bran, essential fatty acids, and nutrients removed—act as simple sugars and also make up a significant part of the diet of many women in Western societies. Many convenience foods (salad dressings, catsup, and relish, to name a few) also contain high levels of both sugar and salt. Some prepackaged desserts and even main courses sold in natural food stores are highly sugared, too, although they are sweetened with fructose, maple syrup, and honey. With sugar so predominant in many foods, it is no wonder sugar addiction is so common in our society among people of all ages. Many people eat sweets as a way to cope with their frustrations and upsets. Statistically, the average American eats more than 120 pounds of sugar per year.

This dietary sugar is eventually metabolized to its simplest form in the body, glucose. Glucose is essential for all cellular processes, since it is the major source of fuel that our cells use to generate energy. However, when we flood our body with too much sugar, it is overwhelmed and cannot process the sugar effectively. This excessive intake can be a major trigger for blood sugar imbalances, food cravings, PMS symptoms, and anxiety symptoms.

It happens like this: unlike simple carbohydrates such as whole grains, beans, and peas, which digest and release sugar slowly, food based on sugar and white flour break down quickly in the digestive tract. Glucose is released rapidly into the blood, and from there is absorbed by the cells of the body to satisfy their energy needs. To handle this overload, the pancreas must release large amounts of insulin. This is the hormone that helps drive glucose into the cells where it can be used as energy.

Often the pancreas releases a flood of insulin, more than the body requires. As a result, the blood sugar level goes from too high to too low, resulting in the "roller coaster" of energy you typically see in hypoglycemia or PMS. You initially feel "high" after eating sugar, followed by a rapid crash. (Excessive amounts of stress also use up glucose rapidly and can cause similar symptoms.) When your blood sugar level falls too low, you begin to feel anxious, jittery, "spacey," and confused because your brain is deprived of its necessary fuel. To remedy this situation, the adrenal glands release hormones which cause your liver to pump stored sugar into your blood stream. While the adrenal hormones boost the blood sugar level, they unfortunately also increase arousal symptoms and anxiety. Thus, both the initial brain deprivation of glucose and the adrenal gland's response to restore the glucose levels can intensify symptoms of anxiety and panic in susceptible women.

Several studies have shown the relationship between the overindulgence of simple sugars and resulting PMS symptoms. One study published in the *Journal of Applied Nutrition* found that women with PMS symptoms had a 50 percent higher sugar intake than normal volunteers. Another study published in the *American Journal of Psychiatry* found that women with PMS were more likely than others to crave sweets and experience emotional symptoms premenstrually.

With continued overuse of sugar, the pancreas eventually wears out and is no longer able to clear sugar from the blood efficiently. The blood sugar level rises and diabetes mellitus is the result. This tendency towards diabetes or high blood sugar levels increases dramatically after menopause. Studies show that more than 50 percent of Americans have blood sugar imbalances by the age of sixty-five.

Excess sugar can worsen the anxiety, irritability, and nervous tension that many women feel as they transition into menopause. One study even suggests that a diet high in sugar can impair liver function and affect the liver's ability to metabolize estrogen. Highly sugared foods also promote tooth decay and gum disease. Many women, however, are addicted to sugar and have a difficult time controlling their intake once they start eating sugary foods like cookies and candy.

The excessive use of sugar has further detrimental effects on the body. Like caffeine, sugar depletes the body's B-complex vitamins and minerals, thereby increasing nervous tension, anxiety, and irritability. Too much sugar also intensifies tiredness by causing vasoconstriction (the narrowing of the diameter of blood vessels) and putting stress on the nervous system in women with chronic fatigue. Candida feeds on sugar, so overindulging in this high-stress food aggravates chronic candida infections. Many women with chronic candida overgrowth notice a worsening of emotional symptoms like depression and nervous tension. Sugar (as well as caffeine, alcohol, flavor enhancers, and white flour) also appears to be a trigger for binge eating and even bulimia. In fact, research has shown that when women switch from a diet high in sugar to a sugar-free, high-nutrient diet, their food addictive behavior tends to cease. After making the switch from a high-sugar diet, women tend to lose or maintain weight more easily and gain relief from the pattern of craving and bingeing. In one small study of 20 women, the women on a nutrient-rich diet (free of sugar and other high-stress foods) were able to remain binge-free for two and a half years.

Because sugar is so deleterious to good health, it is best for menopausal women to avoid sugar entirely or limit its use to small amounts on occasion. It is easy to substitute for sugar in recipes by using fruit, sugar substitutes like aspartame (if you can tolerate them without side effects), or smaller amounts of more concentrated sweeteners. Also, become a label reader. When canned and bottled foods like salad dressings, soft drinks, and baked beans have sugar near the top of the list of ingredients, the product probably contains too much sugar. If so, find alternatives that don't use sugar or only in very small amounts. If you crave sweets, keep fresh or dried fruits in the house like apples, bananas, or dried figs. Whole grain snacks can be a more healthful choice, too. A good example is an oatmeal cookie or a bran muffin sweetened with fruit juice. You can use whole fruit and whole grain products in small amounts to satisfy your craving for sweets; as an added benefit, they provide many essential nutrients. Instead of disrupting your mood and energy levels, these foods may actually have a healthful effect on the body. If you have hypoglycemia or PMS-related blood sugar imbalances, you should avoid simple sugar entirely. Instead, eat a good amount of complex carbohydrates such as whole grains, potatoes, fruits, and vegetables. The sugar in these foods is digested slowly and released gradually into the blood circulation. Thus, the amount of sugar released never overwhelms the body's ability to process it. For even more blood sugar control, combine complex carbohydrates with protein and essential fatty acids. I usually recommend that patients eat foods like tuna fish on toast, and sesame or almond butter on rice cakes.

In an attempt to reduce table sugar intake and other sweeteners, many women will resort to using artificial sweeteners. Unlike natural sweeteners, which are extracted from real food and do have nutritive value as sources of energy, artificial sweeteners are strictly products of the laboratory. They have a sweet taste but no inherent nutrient value.

Two artificial sweeteners—aspartame and saccharin—currently dominate the American market. Aspartame is the newer of the two. It is manufactured from phenylalanine and aspartic acid, two different amino acids. Though many women tolerate aspartame well, some do not. Many of my PMS patients or patients with generalized anxiety or food allergies find that aspartame intensifies anxiety and nervous tension, worsens "the jitters,"and even can trigger a rapid heartbeat. In addition, people with phenylketonuria (PKU) are born without the enzyme needed to metabolize phenylalanine. They cannot digest the large amounts of phenylalanine found in the myriad of artificially sweetened soft drinks, desserts, and dietetic foods that are ubiquitous in our society (as well as food naturally high in phenylalanine). People born with this genetic problem find that phenylalanine ingestion triggers headaches, dizziness, mood swings, and other symptoms. On the positive side, however, aspartame is probably the safest artificial sweetener on the market. Since it is 200 times sweeter than table sugar, people need very little to achieve desired culinary results.

The other artificial sweetener currently on the market is saccharin. While it has been used for many decades, much research suggests that it may be mildly carcinogenic in animals. Saccharin, too, is quite sweet and, in fact, is 300 times sweeter than sugar (although it does have a slightly bitter aftertaste). Saccharin contains no calories whatsoever, and, until the advent of aspartame, was the main artificial sweetener used by millions of Americans trying to lose weight. However, because of the health concerns regarding its use, the U.S. Food and Drug Administration (FDA) has been trying to remove it from the marketplace for many years. As of this writing, it can still be purchased freely in most supermarkets.

A third type of sweetener called cyclamates was actually banned from the market in 1969. Packaged under the brand name Sucaryl, it was a very popular type of artificial sweetener used throughout the 1960s. Laboratory tests found that high dosages of cyclamates produced bladder cancer in research animals.

No artificial sweetener currently on the market is without drawbacks or potential health hazards. It is best to use utilize natural sweeteners in small amounts if you are concerned about potential side effects of artificial sweetners or if you find that you do not tolerate them at all.

Negative Effects of Sugar

Anxiety and panic episodes
Bulimia
Candida
Chronic fatigue
Diabetes mellitus
Food addiction
Hypoglycemia
Loss of B vitamins and
   minerals
Menopausal mood and
   low-energy symptoms
Obesity
PMS-related emotional
   symptoms and food
   cravings
Tooth decay and gum disease

Common Food Sources of Sugar

Beverages: soft drinks, mixed sweet drinks
Convenience foods: salad dressing, catsup, relish
Desserts: cookies, candies, cakes, pies, ice cream
White flour products: pasta, bread, crackers, pastries

Salt

Many foods like cheese and meat, as well as salt-flavored condiments such as table salt and monosodium glutamate (MSG), generally contain large amounts of sodium. Sodium is one of the body's major minerals. It is found primarily in the body's extracellular compartment and in the fluids within the vascular compartments. The rest is stored within the genes. Along with potassium, the primary intracellular mineral, sodium helps to regulate the cell's water balance. Water tends to accumulate in areas where sodium collects. Thus, an over-abundance of sodium in relationship to the body's potassium levels can lead to edema, bloating, and even some cases of high blood pressure.

During the active reproductive years, ingesting too much salt can worsen premenstrual bloating, fluid retention, and breast tenderness during the week or two prior to the onset of menstruation. It can also worsen the dull aching pain that can accompany menstrual cramps at the beginning of the menstrual period. With the onset of menopause, excess sodium intake is a risk factor for many other health problems like cardiovascular disease and hypertension. Women at high risk for developing these problems should certainly curtail their sodium intake.

Bloating and fluid retention are very common in menopausal women. Fluid retention often adds to the excess pounds that can be so irksome; many women complain that they gain 10 to 15 pounds after menopause and that the weight is very difficult to lose, even with dieting and exercise. Of even greater concern is the fact that excess sodium is a risk factor for osteoporosis, since it accelerates calcium loss from the body.

Besides regular table salt, MSG, another sodium-containing flavor enhancer, has been implicated in health problems. MSG is often used in food preparation in Chinese restaurants. It is also a common ingredient in many commercial seasonings, meats, condiments, and oven-baked goods. Besides causing headaches and anxiety episodes, this chemical seems to worsen my patients' food cravings and food addictions.

Unfortunately, avoiding salt and MSG in the American diet, like sugar, takes some work because it is so prevalent. In fact, salt and sugar are often found together in large amounts in frozen, canned, cured, and processed foods. Many of us eat so much salt (far beyond the recommended 2000 mg or one teaspoon per day) that our palates have become jaded. Many people feel that food tastes too bland without the addition of salt. Fast foods such as hamburgers, hot dogs, French fries, pizza, and tacos are loaded with salt and saturated fats. Common processed foods such as soups, potato chips, cheese, olives, pickles, salad dressings, and catsup (to name only a few) are also heavily laden with salt. One frozen-food entree can contribute as much as one-half teaspoon of salt to your daily intake. And if this was not bad enough, many people use the salt shaker liberally in their own cooking and seasoning.

Fortunately, there are many other seasoning options available that are much better for your health. For flavoring, use garlic, basil, oregano, and other herbs. The fresh foods that we eat such as vegetables, grains, legumes, and meat contain all the salt we need, so added table salt isn't necessary. As with sugar, it is important that you read the labels before you buy bottled, canned, or frozen food. Don't buy a product if salt is listed as a main ingredient (near the top of the label). Many brands in the health food stores and supermarkets now distribute foods labeled "no salt added" or "reduced salt." Be sure to buy these rather than the high-salt foods. If you are sensitive to MSG, be sure to check labels of bottled salad dressings and sauces to make sure that it is not an ingredient. Also, eat at Chinese restaurants that advertise "No MSG" in their ads or in

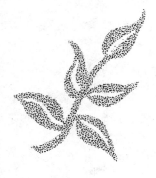

their windows. Many restaurants are aware of the reactions that people have to MSG, so they forego using it in food preparation. Be knowledgeable about the salt substitutes available in natural food stores like miso (flavored soy paste of Japanese origin) or Bragg's Liquid Amino Acids. These and other foods impart a salty taste with less sodium. Also, eat plenty of fresh fruits and vegetables since they are excellent sources of potassium and other essential nutrients. Potassium helps balance the sodium in the body and regulate the blood pressure to keep it at normal levels.

Red Meat, Eggs, and Dairy Products

Red meat (such as beef, pork, and lamb), eggs, and dairy products (such as butter, cream, milk, yogurt, and ice cream) are the main sources of saturated fats in the typical American diet. These fats are solid at room temperature and tend to be more stable and become rancid more slowly than the healthier polyunsaturated fats. Unlike polyunsaturated fats (found primarily in vegetable sources such as raw seeds and nuts, green leafy vegetables, and fish), saturated fats can contribute to such common health problems as heart disease, cancer, obesity, and arthritis. Unfortunately, 40 percent of the calories in the American diet come from these unhealthy, meat-derived saturated fats. The American breakfast of eggs, bacon, milk, toast and butter, as well as dinner choices like hot dogs, hamburgers, pizza, and milk shakes, are loaded with saturated fats.

During the active reproductive years, a diet high in saturated fat increases the risk of menstrual cramps, PMS, ovarian cysts, benign breast disease, endometriosis, fibroid tumors of the uterus, heavy menstrual bleeding, and other female health problems. Changing the diet can be difficult for women because meat and dairy products have traditionally been touted as important food groups. Most women consider them the mainstay of their diets, consuming large amounts of cheese, yogurt, milk, cottage cheese, eggs, and meat. Yet meat and dairy products are the main dietary sources of arachidonic acid, the fat that your body uses to produce the series-2 prostaglandin hormones. These hormones are the main culprits implicated in causing the painful menstrual cramps experienced by 50 percent of all younger American women. In my practice, I have seen the severity of menstrual cramps decrease by as much as one-third to one-half within one menstrual cycle when women completely eliminated these foods from their diet. Also, the high-salt content of dairy products increases the bloating and fluid retention usually seen one to two weeks before the onset of menstruation in women suffering from PMS. In postmenopausal women, arachidonic acid-derived PGE 2 increases the risk of many health problems emerging during the later years. It actually promotes platelet aggregation or clumping, thereby initiating potentially dangerous clot formation. It also causes inflammation and fluid retention, which can predispose postmenopausal women towards arthritis and high blood pressure.

Besides increasing the levels of the harmful series-2 prostaglandin hormones, the regular use of dairy products, red meat, and eggs also increases estrogen levels in the body. In fact, the blood estrogen levels found in omnivores differs strikingly from those of vegetarian women who eat a low-fat, high-fiber diet. Specifically, omnivores have 50 percent higher blood estrogen levels and only one-third to one-half the blood estrogen excretion rates of vegetarian women. Studies conducted at Tufts University Medical School explained why this is the case. Researchers found that under optimal dietary conditions, large amounts of dietary fiber (normally found in fruits, vegetables, grains, and legumes) bind with estrogen, aiding its excretion from the body in the bowel movements. This helps to regulate the blood estrogen levels and keep them from rising too high. Predictably, women eating a high-fat, low-fiber diet have higher blood levels of estrogen. Fat promotes the growth of intestinal bacteria that can act chemically on estrogen metabolites, reactivating them so that they can be reabsorbed back into the body. Elevated levels of estrogen can worsen a variety of female complaints, including PMS, fibroid tumors of the uterus, heavy menstrual bleeding, endometriosis, and benign breast disease.

As women reach midlife, the use of meat, eggs, and dairy products can promote a host of other health problems. Saturated fat tends to increase the cholesterol levels in the blood, particularly the high-risk, low-density lipoproteins that initiate plaque formation in the blood vessels. Plaque formation can eventually lead to heart attacks and strokes. In contrast, the "good" fats derived from fish and vegetable sources can actually prevent heart attacks by reducing the tendency for the blood to clot. A high-saturated fat diet can also lead to obesity in women of all ages. Menopausal women are particularly at risk since, as their metabolism slows down with age, they burn calories less efficiently. One gram of fat contains 9 calories versus the 4 calories contained in one gram of protein or carbohydrate. As a result, fatty foods tend to be much higher in calories per unit weight. While saturated fats do provide the body with a concentrated source of energy, very few of us need these extra calories. Instead of burning the fat for energy, we tend to store it in our cells as excess pounds.

A high-fat, low-fiber diet is also associated with colon cancer, prostate cancer in men, and some breast cancer in women. As mentioned earlier, a high-fat diet promotes the conversion of estrogen metabolites by anaerobic bacteria in the intestinal tract to forms of estrogen that can be easily reabsorbed back into the body. This elevates the blood estrogen level with types of estrogen that may increase some women's susceptibility to breast cancer. In contrast, lowering the amount of dietary fat while increasing the amount of high-fiber foods in the diet can help reduce the risk of hormone-related cancers in women.

Many American women base their meals on meat and dairy entrees like steaks, chops, meat sandwiches, cheese sandwiches, and yogurt. Unfortunately, large amounts of meat-based protein can increase the risk of osteoporosis. Meat protein is acidic; when a woman eats meat in excessive amounts, her body must buffer the acid load that meat creates. One way the body accomplishes this is by dissolving the bones. The calcium and other minerals released from the bones helps restore the body's acid-alkaline balance. (This process does not occur with dairy products which already contain calcium.) One study comparing the incidence of osteoporosis in meat-eating women (omnivores) with that among vegetarians found a dramatic difference in bone density after age sixty. Between the ages of sixty and eighty-nine, vegetarian women lost 18 percent of their bone mass, but meat-eating women lost 35 percent of their bone mass. Quite a striking difference. Other studies show that the amount of protein eaten can make a difference in calcium levels. Protein intake over three ounces a day causes loss of the calcium from the urinary tract. This has been found to be true even in low-risk groups such as young, healthy males.

Finally, meat, dairy products, and saturated oils (like coconut and palm-kernel oil) are difficult to digest. As women age, they secrete less hydrochloric acid and fewer of the digestive enzymes needed for fat and protein breakdown in the intestinal tract. In one study, 40 percent of postmenopausal women lacked hydrochloric acid. Without sufficient hydrochloric acid, calcium and iron absorption become more difficult. For women of all ages with chronic tiredness, a meat- and dairy-based diet can aggravate these symptoms. This is because the body must use so much energy to break these foods down before they can be absorbed, assimilated, and finally utilized. All parts of dairy products are difficult to digest—the fat, the protein, and the milk sugar. Digesting dairy products demands hydrochloric acids, enzymes, and fat emulsifiers, which a fatigued woman may not produce in sufficient quantities. Eggs and meat protein are equally difficult to digest for a chronically tired woman.

Dairy foods can also aggravate other health problems. Many women are specifically allergic to dairy products, and dairy products intensify allergy symptoms in general. Besides fatigue, users of dairy products often complain of allergy-based nasal congestion, sinus swelling, and postnasal drip. They might also suffer from digestive problems such as bloating, gas, and bowel changes, which intensify with menstruation. This intolerance to dairy products can hamper the absorption and assimilation of the calcium these products contain. Also, clinical studies have shown that dairy products decrease iron absorption in anemic women.

Women concerned about losing calcium by eliminating dairy products from their diet can choose many other food sources of calcium. These include beans and peas, soybeans, sesame seeds, soup stock made from chicken or fish bones, and green leafy vegetables. A delicious potato-based milk called Vegelicious, as well as soy milks and nut milk are excellent substitutes for food preparation. These nondairy milks are readily available at health food stores, and many of them are calcium fortified. You can also take a supplement containing calcium, magnesium, and vitamin D to make sure your intake is sufficient.

For optimal protein intake, your diet should emphasize

whole grains, beans and peas, seeds and nuts, and fish high in the beneficial Omega-3 fatty acids. Red meat and dairy products are best eliminated or eaten occasionally in small portions. This is truly an optimal diet for most women, emphasizing high-nutrient content, low-stress foods, and easy digestibility.

If you feel the need to eat meat other than fish, poultry is the best option. Serve poultry broiled or roasted and without the skin. Avoid heavy sauces or dressings. Always buy lean cuts and trim off all visible fat. Fish and poultry should be eaten more frequently than beef, pork, or lamb, which are higher in fat. American dinners traditionally center around a large piece of meat or fish, with small servings of grain and vegetables as side dishes. For women who want to enjoy optimal health throughout their lives, I recommend reversing this ratio. Keep your meat portions small (3 oz) and fill up with a variety of other nutritious side dishes. Try to buy meat from organic range-fed sources. This type of meat has undergone less exposure to pesticides, antibiotics, and hormones. Most people eat much more meat protein than necessary. In fact, if you find meat difficult to digest, you might be deficient in hydrochloric acid, a digestive enzyme normally found in the stomach. Try taking a small amount of hydrochloric acid (available in tablet form in natural foods stores) with every meat-containing meal to see if your digestion improves.

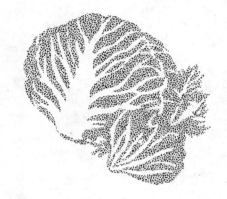

Female Problems Aggravated by Red Meat, Eggs, and Dairy Products

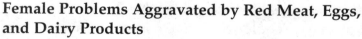

Benign breast disease	Menopause
Breast cancer	Menstrual cramps
Endometriosis	Osteoporosis
Fibroid tumors of the uterus	Ovarian cysts
Heavy menstrual bleeding	PMS

General Health Problems Aggravated by Red Meat, Eggs, and Dairy Products

Cancer of the prostate   Constipation
Cardiovascular disease   Digestive complaints
Chronic fatigue   Food allergies
Colon cancer   Hypertension

Foods High in Saturated Fat

Beef   Eggs   Pork
Butter   Ice cream   Sour cream
Cheese   Lamb   Yogurt
Coconut oil   Milk
Cream cheese   Palm oil

Margarine

Margarine is a golden-yellow solid spread that has been touted for many decades as a healthier alternative to butter. It is manufactured of polyunsaturated vegetable oils that are altered chemically by saturating their carbon bonds with hydrogen. Hydrogenation changes the liquid vegetable oils to a solid. As a result, it can be used like butter on toast, rolls, and other foods. Hydrogenation also renders the oils more stable, so they are less perishable and have a longer shelf life.

The "margarine is healthy" campaign has been very effective in terms of sales. People who were concerned about their cholesterol levels and risk of heart attack abandoned butter and dramatically increased margarine use. In fact, by 1980, margarine consumption was almost triple that of butter. Hydrogenated and partially-hydrogenated oils are ubiquitous, used in all types of fast-food products and processed foods. These include crackers, snack foods, salad oils, and cooking oils, to name but a few types of products.

Are the health claims made for margarine actually true? A number of studies have turned up troubling data on this subject. While it is true that margarine contains no cholesterol, the process of hydrogenation changes not only the physical form of the oils, but alters the way they are metabolized by the body. Once vegetable oils are hydrogenated, they are no longer polyunsaturated. In fact, with hydrogenation, the beneficial structure of the essential fatty acids is altered or destroyed. As a result, the final margarine product is much lower in essential fatty acids. Most of the beneficial oils have been changed to a form called trans-fatty acids. These trans-fatty acids tend to predominate in margarine, with some samples containing as much as 60 percent of their oils in this altered form.

Trans-fatty acids behave differently than the natural oils from which they were derived. They burn more slowly than natural oils and interfere with their function. Trans-fatty acids also tend to concentrate in the heart. Ominously, recent studies show that people eating four or more teaspoons per day of margarine actually have a significantly increased risk of cardiovascular disease. In one study reported in the *New England Journal of Medicine*, the trans-fatty acids in margarine were found to increase LDL cholesterol. This is the type of cholesterol associated with an increased risk of heart attacks. Trans-fatty acids were also found to lower the beneficial and protective HDL cholesterol levels. Other studies have shown that trans-fatty acids also increase the level of triglycerides, another risk factor for cardiovascular disease.

Another drawback of margarine is that its high water content continues to alter its chemical structure while it is on the supermarket shelf. This degrades the product further.

What is the solution? Ideally, people in our society should decrease their intake, both margarine and butter. With 40 percent of the average American diet composed of fats, intake of margarine should be sharply curtailed. For those women who want to continue to use fats in food preparation, the amount should be decreased significantly. Steaming, roasting, broiling, and other preparation techniques that are fat-free should be favored over frying and sautéing in large quantities of oil. When cooking with oil, often a small amount will work just as well. Instead of using margarine as a spread for toast, rolls, or other grain products, use fresh fruit preserves or raw seed and nut butters that have their natural oils intact. Try olive oil as a topping instead of margarine; it is delicious on bread and toast. Avoid fast-food outlets since they tend to use partially hydrogenated oils in much of their food preparation. Also, read labels carefully when you buy convenience foods and processed foods in the supermarket. If they contain hydrogenated oil, you are better off buying a safer substitute that contains natural oil, or no oils.

Part II

Vitamins, Minerals, and Herbs for Female Health Problems

CHAPTER 3

PMS and
Menstrual Migraines

*P*MS is one of the most common female health complaints during active reproductive years, affecting women from their teenage years to their fifties. In fact, one third to one-half of women in America in this age group are estimated to suffer from PMS (with 10 percent having severe symptoms). This translates into as many as ten to fifteen million women.

The symptoms of PMS typically occur after midcycle and can last from a few days prior to the onset of menstruation to as long as ten to fourteen days per month. For most, symptoms begin to decline fairly rapidly once menstruation begins. For women with moderate to severe symptoms, this can mean time each month with decreased work productivity and a diminished quality of life.

More than 150 symptoms of PMS have been documented. Some of these symptoms occur frequently. Among the most common symptoms are anxiety, irritability, mood swings, fatigue, depression, migraine headaches, food cravings (especially salt and sugar), poor concentration, dizziness, fluid retention and bloating, breast tenderness, and acne. Quite often a woman will have a combination of these symptoms.

Studies have linked the causes of PMS to several dozen hormonal and chemical imbalances including estrogen-progesterone imbalances, prolactin (milk release hormone) sensitivity, nutritional imbalances, and neurotransmitter (chemicals that transfer messages from one part of the brain to the other) imbalances. Hormonal inbalances, however, have been specifically linked to menstrual migraines. All of these hormones regulate fluid balance and relaxation and constriction of blood vessels and muscles. When they are out of balance, headaches may occur.

While PMS is treated by physicians with antianxiety medication, antidepressants, birth control pills, and diuretics, lifestyle modification can play a significant role in symptom relief and prevention. This includes dietary modification, the use of nutritional supplements, stress reduction techniques, and exercise.

Vitamins and Minerals for PMS

Vitamin A. In several studies of women taking very high doses, vitamin A (greater than 100,000 IU per day) was found to be effective in relieving their PMS symptoms. Physical symptoms, particularly bloating and fluid retention, appeared to respond better than emotional ones. PMS-related acne has also been shown to benefit from vitamin A use.

Unfortunately, there is a drawback to taking vitamin A in such high doses. Vitamin A, an oil-soluble vitamin derived from fish liver, tends to accumulate in the human liver. When taken in high doses, it can build to toxic levels in the liver, causing irritation, abdominal pain, and headaches. Symptoms of vitamin A toxicity can include headaches and liver irritation. High doses of vitamin A (greater than 25,000 IU per day) should be monitored by a physician.

Fortunately, an alternative source of vitamin A is available from fruits and vegetables. This is the provitamin A called beta carotene. Beta carotene is converted to vitamin A in our liver and intestines as needed by the body. It can be used safely in high doses (50,000—100,000 IU per day) by most people. In fact, it is relatively easy to take doses of beta carotene at this level through diet alone. For example, one sweet potato or one cup of carrot juice each contains approximately 20,000 IU of beta carotene.

Vitamin B complex. This vitamin complex consists of eleven separate B vitamins which are often found together in food. In many cases they participate in the same chemical reactions in the body, often needing to work together for the best results.

Research conducted at UCLA Medical School shows that a lack of sufficient B complex can worsen the emotional symptoms of PMS—anxiety, irritability, mood swings, and depression. Conversely, adequate intake of these nutrients can help to calm the mood and provide a stable and constant source of energy.

B-complex vitamins also help regulate mood by facilitating carbohydrate metabolism and the cellular conversion of glucose to usable energy (ATP). Supplementation with B vitamins also helps to decrease sugar and chocolate cravings in women with PMS. When they are deficient, the liver is unable to efficiently perform its role as the body's chief detoxifying organ. This role includes the inactivation of estrogen. Excessive levels of estrogen act as a brain stimulant, worsening symptoms of anxiety and nervous tension. It can also worsen fluid and salt retention, thereby triggering menstrual migraines.

Deficiencies of individual B vitamins also increase anxiety and stress. Pantothenic acid (vitamin B_5) is needed for healthy adrenal function. High emotional stress, typically seen with PMS, triggers the fight-or-flight alarm response in the body, which includes excessive output of adrenal hormones. A deficiency of pantothenic acid can intensify this response.

Pyridoxine (vitamin B_6) also affects moods through its important role in the conversion of linoleic acid to gamma linolenic acid (GLA) in the production of the beneficial series-1 prostaglandins. Prostaglandins are hormonelike chemicals that have a relaxant effect on both mood and smooth muscle tissue. Lack of these relaxant hormones has been linked to PMS-related anxiety and stress-related problems like irritable bowel syndrome and migraine headaches, including those experienced during menstruation. The use of the birth control pill, a common treatment for PMS, menstrual cramps, and irregularity, decreases vitamin B_6 levels. Paradoxically, however, PMS-like symptoms can occur as a side effect of hormone use, partially due to B_6 deficiency. B_6 supplementation may help reduce these symptoms. B_6 can be safely used in doses up to 300 mg. Doses above this level can be neurotoxic and should be avoided.

Lack of B_6 may also increase anxiety symptoms directly through its effect on the nervous system. B_6 is needed for the conversion of the amino acid tryptophan to serotonin, an important neurotransmitter. Serotonin regulates sleep, and when it is deficient, insomnia occurs—a condition often seen in anxious women. Serotonin levels also strongly affect mood and social behavior. Both B_6 and food sources of tryptophan such as almonds, pumpkin seeds, sesame seeds, and certain other protein-containing foods are necessary for adequate serotonin production.

In summary, the entire range of B vitamins is needed to provide nutritional support to combat anxiety and stress symptoms. Because B vitamins are water soluble, the body cannot readily store them. Thus, B vitamins must be taken in the diet daily. Women who are anxious and experience significant stress should eat foods high in B vitamins and take vitamin supplements. Good sources of most B vitamins include brewer's yeast (which many women cannot digest readily), liver, whole grain germ and bran, beans, peas, and nuts. B_{12} is found mainly in animal foods. Women following a vegan diet (a vegetarian diet containing no dairy products or eggs) should take particular care to add supplemental vitamin B_{12} to their diets.

Vitamin C. An extremely important antistress nutrient, vitamin C that can help decrease the fatigue symptoms that often accompany excessive levels of PMS-related anxiety and stress. It is needed for the production of adrenal gland hormones. When the fight-or-flight pattern is activated in response to stress, these hormones become depleted. Larger amounts of vitamin C in the diet are needed when stress levels are high. In one research study testing 411 dentists and their spouses, scientists found a clear relationship between the lack of vitamin C and the presence of fatigue.

The best natural sources of vitamin C are fruits and vegetables. Vitamin C is water soluble, thus it is not stored in the body. Women with anxiety and stress should replenish their vitamin C supply daily.

Vitamin E. In one controlled study, women with anxiety, irritability, mood swings, depression, and food cravings noted symptom relief with addition of 150 to 600 IU of vitamin E daily. Symptom relief ranged as high as 38 percent, a significant amount to be attributed to the use of only one nutrient. A study of PMS-related breast tenderness also found vitamin E to be an effective treatment. Daily doses of 300 to 600 IU were given for three months. Most of the subjects noted moderate to complete relief of breast discomfort. Many women in the study noted a reduction in the size of their breast cysts. Vitamin E is also a natural muscle relaxant and antispasmodic. As a result, it may help in preventing menstrual migraines.

The best natural sources of vitamin E are wheat germ oil,

walnut oil, soybean oil, and other grain and seed oils. I generally recommend that women with menopause- and PMS-related anxiety take vitamin E supplements of between 400 to 2000 IU per day. Women with hypertension, diabetes, or bleeding problems should start on a much lower dose of vitamin E (100 IU per day). If you have any of these conditions, ask your physician about the advisability of taking these supplements. Any increase in dosage should be made slowly and monitored carefully. Otherwise, vitamin E tends to be extremely safe and is commonly used by millions of people.

Magnesium. Researchers at UCLA Medical School found that not only is vitamin B complex important for relief of PMS symptoms, but that magnesium also plays an important therapeutic role. Studies found that red blood cell magnesium levels are lower in women with PMS during the time of the month when they are more irritable, tired, and depressed.

There are several reasons why magnesium deficiency can aggravate PMS. First of all, the body requires adequate levels of magnesium in order to maintain energy and vitality. Women suffering from excessive levels of anxiety experience greater stress on the body and depleted energy. The body needs magnesium in order to produce ATP, the end product of the conversion of food to usable energy by the body's cells. ATP is the universal energy currency that the body uses to run hundreds of thousands of chemical reactions. The digestive system can efficiently extract this energy from food only in the presence of magnesium, oxygen, and other nutrients. When magnesium is deficient, ATP production falls and the body forms lactic acid instead. Researchers have linked excessive accumulation of lactic acid with anxiety and irritability symptoms.

Magnesium is also needed to facilitate both the conversion of linoleic acid, an essential fatty acid, to gamma linolenic acid

(GLA) and the conversion of GLA to the beneficial, relaxant prostaglandin hormones. Stimulating production of these hormones helps to reduce the anxiety and mood swing symptoms of PMS, eating disorders, and agoraphobia. Several studies have found that magnesium deficiency may predispose a woman to menstrual migraines. In one study, magnesium nitrate was given to 192 women one week premenstrually and during the first two days of menstruation. Nervous tension was relieved in 89 percent of the women studied. They also noted relief of headaches, breast tenderness, and weight gain. Magnesium is needed for adrenal health. This is noteworthy since the adrenal gland helps to mediate physiological stress in the body.

Magnesium supplements can also benefit women with PMS-related insomnia. When taken before bedtime, magnesium helps calm the mood and induce restful sleep. Food sources of magnesium include green leafy vegetables, beans and peas, raw nuts and seeds, tofu, avocados, raisins, dried figs, millet, and other grains.

Essential Fatty Acids. A number of studies from Canada and England using essential fatty acids (specifically, evening primrose oil) have shown significant benefits for relief of PMS symptoms. In 60 to 70 percent of the women studied, evening primrose oil supplements decreased symptoms of emotional upset, mood swings, and breast tenderness. Essential fatty acids are the raw materials from which prostaglandins are made. Prostaglandins have muscle-relaxant and blood vessel-relaxant properties that can significantly reduce fluid retention in the kidneys and may also help to prevent migraine headaches.

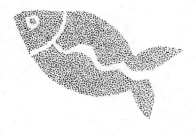

Linoleic acid (Omega-6 family) and linolenic acid (Omega-3 family), the two essential fatty acids, are derived from specific food sources in our diet: raw seeds and nuts, and certain fish including salmon, mackerel, sardines, halibut, and trout. Linoleic and linolenic acids are not made by the body and must be consumed daily, through food or supplements. Even if the diet contains significant amounts of fatty acids, some women may lack the ability to convert them efficiently to the muscle-relaxant prostaglandins. This is particularly true of linoleic acid, which must be converted to gamma linolenic acid (GLA) on its way to becoming the series-1 prostaglandin.

The conversion of linoleic acid to GLA, and the reaction which creates the beneficial prostaglandins, requires the presence of magnesium, zinc, vitamin B_6, vitamin C, and niacin. When women are deficient in these nutrients, their bodies can't make the chemical conversions effectively. A diet high in cholesterol, processed oils, and alcohol makes the fatty acid conversion to the series-1 prostaglandin difficult to achieve. Other factors that impede prostaglandin production include emotional stress, allergies, and eczema. In women with these risk factors, less than 1 percent of linoleic acid might be converted to GLA. The rest of the fatty acids might be used as an energy source, but they will not be able to play a role in relieving anxiety and stress symptoms.

Evening primrose oil, borage oil, and black currant oil are the most common supplemental sources of essential fatty acids for the treatment of PMS. All three oils contain high levels of GLA, allowing the body to circumvent the difficult conversion process of linoleic acid to GLA. The best food sources of essential fatty acids are raw flax seed oil and pumpkin seed oil, which contain high levels of linoleic and linolenic fatty acids. Both the seeds and their pressed oils can be used and should be absolutely fresh and unspoiled. As mentioned earlier, these oils become rancid rapidly when exposed to light and air (oxygen), and they need to be packed in special opaque containers and kept refrigerated.

My special favorite is fresh flax seed oil—so golden, rich, and delicious. It is extremely high in linoleic and linolenic acids, which comprise approximately 80 percent of its total content. Flax oil has a wonderful flavor and can be used as a butter replacement on many foods such as mashed potatoes, air-popped popcorn, steamed broccoli, cauliflower, carrots, and bread. Flax oil (and all other essential oils) should never be heated or used in cooking, as heat affects the special chemical properties of these oils. Instead, add these oils as a flavoring to foods that have been already cooked.

Herbs for Relief of PMS

There are many different types of herbs that help relieve PMS, including:

Sedative and Relaxant Herbs. Herbs such as valerian root, passion flower, hops, chamomile, and skullcap have a significant calming and restful effect on the central nervous system. Other emotionally calming herbs include bay, balm, catnip, celery, motherwort, wild cherry, and yarrow. These herbs can be very helpful for women with PMS-related mood swings, anxiety, and irritability. Their mild sedative effect also promotes restful sleep which some women find difficult to attain during the second half of their menstrual cycle.

Passion flower has been found to elevate levels of the neurotransmitter serotonin. A deficiency of serotonin may be a trigger for PMS symptoms. Serotonin is synthesized from tryptophan, an essential amino acid that has been shown in numerous medical studies to initiate restful sleep. Chamomile, an herb that makes a delicate, tasty tea, is a good source of tryptophan. Valerian root has been used extensively in traditional herbal medicine as a sleep inducer and is widely used now both in Europe and the United States as a gentle herbal remedy to help combat insomnia. Unfortunately, valerian has an unpleasant taste and is more palatable when taken in capsule form.

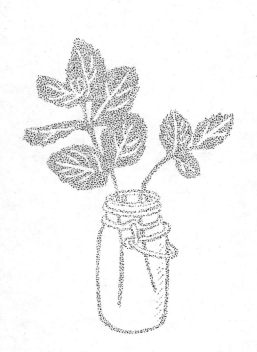

Stimulant Herbs. Some women with PMS find that the symptoms of depression and fatigue occur more often than irritability. For these women, herbs that provide a gentle stimulant effect and build stamina and endurance may be helpful during the premenstrual time (and throughout the month). Herbs such as oat straw, ginger, ginkgo biloba, dandelion root, and Siberian ginseng (eleutherococcus) are known to boost energy and vitality. Some women who have taken these herbs have noted an increased ability to handle stress, as well as improved physical and mental capabilities.

The salutary effects of these herbs may be due to their high levels of essential nutrients. For example, dandelion root contains magnesium, potassium, and vitamin E, while ginkgo is high in bioflavonoids. These essential nutrients help relieve fatigue, depression, PMS, and hot flashes, and they increase resistance to infections. Oat straw has been used to relieve fatigue and weakness, especially when there is an emotional cause.

Siberian ginseng and ginger have been important traditional medicines in Japan, China and other countries for thousands of years. They are reputed to increase longevity and decrease fatigue and weakness.

Bioflavonoid and Other Phytoestrogen-Containing Plants. Bioflavonoids and other sources of plant estrogen may be helpful in relieving PMS-related anxiety and mood swings. This is due to the fact that they have weak estrogenic activity (1/50,000 the strength of a drug dose of estrogen), and can actually interfere with the body's ability to manufacture estrogen. Bioflavonoids can also compete with estrogen manufactured by the body by binding to receptor sites of cells in estrogenic-sensitive tissues like the uterus and breasts. Thus, these estrogenic plants help to regulate and balance estrogen levels in the body. I have found that herbs containing plant estrogen are useful in stabilizing mood. I have also found them to be essential in controlling menstrual migraines. In some women, PMS mood symptoms can be linked to an estrogen-progesterone imbalance. Both of these hormones affect brain chemistry and mood. Progesterone has a sedativelike effect, while estrogen, in excess, can worsen anxiety symptoms. Both hormones also need to be in proper balance to regulate muscle and vascular tone. Besides bioflavonoids, other phytoestrogen plant sources of estrogen and progesterone used in traditional herbology for PMS symptoms include dong quai, black cohosh, blue cohosh, unicorn root, false unicorn root, fennel, anise, sarsaparilla, and wild yam root. The hormonal activities of these plants have been observed in a number of interesting research studies.

Diuretic Herbs. Many herbs act as mild diuretic agents, useful in the treatment of PMS by reducing bloating and fluid retention. I often recommend diuretic herbs in the form of mild teas or tinctures, such as buchu, celery, dandelion, horsetail, parsley, nettle, sarsaparilla, and uva ursi. All of the herbs with diuretic action can deplete your potassium stores on a long-term basis, but they are still much milder than prescription diuretics. If you use these herbs to treat PMS-related fluid retention, be sure to eat foods that are high in potassium such as bananas, oranges, raw seeds, nuts, fresh vegetables, and most fruits.

CHAPTER 4

Menstrual Cramps

Menstrual cramps are so common that they are considered a "garden variety" gynecological problem. As many as 50 percent of all women suffer from menstrual cramps, with the highest incidence found in women from teen years to in the early thirties. Ten percent of women in this age group have symptoms so severe that, for a few days each month, they are unable to function optimally at their job, or carry out normal household activities.

Usually menstrual cramps start a day or two before the actual onset of menstruation and begin to diminish significantly within a day after it begins. However, some women notice pain symptoms as far as a week ahead. Menstrual cramps bring different types of pain sensations, varying from viselike pain to dull, aching pain in the pelvic area. Other complaints include low back pain, "drawing sensations" in the inner thighs, nausea, vomiting, diarrhea, abdominal bloating, headaches, faintness, dizziness, and fatigue.

The viselike spasmodic cramping is due to contraction and tightness of the uterine muscle and constriction of the blood vessels that nourish the uterus. Often the surrounding muscles are also tense. This is due to the overproduction by the body of the series-2 prostaglandins (specifically, the E_2 and F_2 Alpha). These chemicals trigger the muscle contractions that cause the actual cramping. As a result, blood circulation and oxygenation in the pelvic area are diminished, so the metabolism of the uterus and pelvic muscles is decreased. Waste products of metabolism, such as lactic acid and carbon dioxide, accumulate, worsening the pain symptoms.

The symptom of aching pelvic pain, which is often accompanied by low back pain and abdominal bloating, tends to be due to the excessive accumulation of fluid and salt. Unlike the viselike spasmodic pain symptom, these dull aching sensations seem to get worse as a woman ages. In many women, the most severe congestive symptoms occur during their thirties and forties. Excessive amounts of estrogen can worsen these symptoms since estrogen increases fluid and salt retention in the body. Excessive salt intake has a similar effect.

While medication, particularly the antiprostaglandin drugs like aspirin, Motrin, Ponstel, Naprosyn, and others can help dramatically in reducing menstrual cramps, the important role of a healthy lifestyle should not be neglected. Regular exercise, particularly aerobic exercise and stretching, can bring improved blood circulation and oxygenation to the pelvic area. Stretching can help keep the pelvic and back muscles flexible. Because cramps can be worse during times of emotional stress, meditation and deep breathing exercises can help release tension and restore a sense of peace and calm. Women with moderate to severe menstrual cramps should decrease their intake of red meat, poultry, and dairy products, which stimulate the body's production of the series-2 prostaglandins. They should also limit their intake of salt, sugar, chocolate, alcohol, and caffeinated beverages. Instead, they should emphasize a diet high in fruits and vegetables as well as whole grains, beans, peas, raw seeds and nuts, and fish.

Vitamins and Minerals for Menstrual Cramps

The following vitamins and minerals should be very helpful for cramps:

Vitamins B_3 and B_6. These vitamins are particularly helpful for menstrual cramps. Niacin, or vitamin B_3, has been shown in clinical research to be effective in relieving 90 percent of menstrual cramps in symptomatic women. The effectiveness of niacin was enhanced with the addition of vitamin C and rutin, a bioflavonoid. Supplementation needs to be started seven to ten days prior to menses to be effective, and the benefits of niacin often remain for several months after stopping its use. An optimal dose range is 25 to 200 mg per day. However, women with preexisting liver disease should use niacin very cautiously.

Vitamin B_6, or pyridoxine, can be used to help regulate symptoms of both congestive and spasmodic dysmenorrhea. Clinical studies have shown a reduction in cramping, fluid retention, weight gain, and fatigue with the use of B_6. An interesting study done in 1978 tested the effectiveness of vitamin B_6 in decreasing cramps. Women were given B_6 daily throughout their menstrual period as well as during the rest of the month. Duration and intensity of their cramps decreased progressively over a four- to six-month period.

Vitamin B_6 is also an important factor in the conversion of linoleic acid to gamma linolenic acid (GLA) in the production of the series-1 prostaglandins. Series-1 prostaglandins have a relaxant effect on uterine muscles, so they can help to reduce cramps. Since vitamin B_6 levels are decreased in women using the birth control pill, a common treatment for both spasmodic dysmenorrhea and endometriosis, they should be supplemented daily. B_6 can be safely taken in doses up to 300 mg. Doses above this level can be neurotoxic and should be avoided.

Vitamin C. Vitamin C helps improve capillary strength and reduce capillary fragility. This is important for menstrual cramps since it permits better flow of nutrients into the tight and contracted uterine muscle and facilitates the flow of waste products out of the uterus. Waste products that worsen cramping and pain, such as lactic acid and carbon dioxide, are more efficiently released from the pelvic region. Vitamin C is also an important antistress vitamin and can help decrease the fatigue and lethargy symptoms that accompany cramps. I recommend that women with cramps take 500 to 3000 mg of vitamin C per day, especially when symptoms occur.

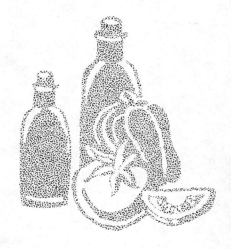

Vitamin E. Vitamin E has been tested clinically as a treatment for spasmodic dysmenorrhea. In one study it was used in doses of 150 IU ten days premenstrual and during the first four days of the menstrual period. In approximately 70 percent of the women tested, it helped to relieve symptoms of menstrual discomfort within two menstrual cycles. The best natural sources of vitamin E are wheat germ oil, walnut oil, soybean oil, and other grain and seed oil sources. I generally recommend that women with cramps take from 400 to 800 IU per day. Women with hypertension and diabetes should start on a much lower dose of vitamin E (100 IU per day). Any increase in dosage should be made slowly and monitored carefully. Otherwise, vitamin E tends to be extremely safe and is commonly used by millions of men and women.

Calcium. This important mineral helps to prevent menstrual cramps by maintaining normal muscle tone. When taken before bed at night, it is also effective in helping to combat insomnia due to menstrual discomfort. Muscles that are calcium-deficient tend to be hyperactive and more likely to cramp. Because the uterus is made up of muscle, it is susceptible to calcium deficiency. Besides its role in promoting normal muscle tone and activity, calcium is also a major structural component of the bones. Unfortunately, calcium deficiency is common in our society. The recommended daily allowance (RDA) for calcium in menstruating women is 800 mg per day and rises to as much as 1500 mg per day in postmenopausal women. The typical American diet supplies only about 450 to 550 mg per day. It's no wonder that so many American women have menstrual cramps and osteoporosis. Food sources of calcium include green leafy vegetables, beans and peas, seeds and nuts, blackstrap molasses, and seafood.

Magnesium. Magnesium has an important effect on the neuromuscular system in reducing menstrual cramps. Like calcium, magnesium reduces muscular hyperactivity. Because of magnesium's importance in glucose metabolism, magnesium deficiency increases menstrual fatigue, dizziness, and fainting. A magnesium deficiency can hinder the normal conversion of food to usable energy. As magnesium is also needed for the conversion of linoleic acid to GLA, a deficiency retards the conversion of essential fatty acids to the series-1 prostaglandins. Magnesium actually optimizes the amount of usable calcium in the system by increasing calcium absorption. Conversely, calcium can interfere with magnesium absorption. It is usually recommended that the diet include half as much magnesium as calcium, or approximately 400 mg per day. Most women get only one-third to one-half of that amount in their daily diet. This puts them at high risk of developing menstrual cramping and pain.

Iron. Women who have iron-deficiency anemia may be more likely to suffer from menstrual cramps because of the diminished oxygen-carrying capability of their red blood cells. One study showed that when iron-deficiency anemia was resolved, menstrual cramping disappeared. Young women in their teens and twenties are not only very prone to iron deficiency, but they are also at the peak age for spasmodic dysmenorrhea. Teenagers are prone to heavier menstrual flows during the first few years after they begin menstruation. Also, teenagers and young women in their twenties often eat an iron-poor diet, full of fat and sugar. The RDA for iron is 15 mg. Food sources of iron include blackstrap molasses, seafood, eggs, liver, vegetables, seeds, nuts, beans, and peas.

Essential Fatty Acids. Essential fatty acids are very important nutrients for the reduction of menstrual cramps. The two essential fatty acids, linoleic acid (found primarily in raw seeds and nuts) and linolenic acid (found primarily in fish such as salmon, trout, sardines, halibut, and mackerel; leafy green vegetables; and a few seeds and nuts), are the raw materials from which prostaglandins are made. The prostaglandins produced from essential fatty acids have muscle-relaxant and blood vessel-relaxant properties that can significantly reduce muscle cramps and tension.

Some women's bodies are unable to convert linoleic acid efficiently to gamma linolenic acid (GLA), which is then converted into necessary prostaglandins.

These are some of the factors that impede prostaglandin production:

- deficiency in vitamins B_6 and C, and magnesium, zinc, and niacin
- diet high in cholesterol, processed oils, and alcohol
- diabetes, allergies, and eczema
- emotional stress

In women with these factors present, less than 1 percent of linoleic acid gets converted to GLA. The other fatty acids in the body can be energy sources, but they will not relieve menstrual cramps.

These women often benefit greatly from taking a GLA supplement such as evening primrose oil, borage oil, or black currant oil. Also, they can consume raw flax seed oil and pumpkin seed oil; these contain high levels of linoleic and linolenic fatty acids. The seeds and their pressed oils should be absolutely fresh and care should be taken not to let these oils become rancid by exposure to light and air (oxygen). Make sure to buy oils packaged in special opaque containers and keep them refrigerated even before opening them.

Herbs for Menstrual Cramps

Following are suggested herbs for menstrual cramps:

Sedative Herbs. These herbs not only have a calming and relaxing effect on women with PMS mood swings and irritability, but are also useful for women with menstrual cramps. Valerian root, passion flower, hops, and chamomile calm the central nervous system. They promote muscle relaxation as well as a sense of well-being. With their mild sedative effect, they also help provide restful sleep, a state that is difficult to achieve when a woman is suffering from menstrual pain. Passion flower has been found to elevate levels of serotonin, which is synthesized from tryptophan, an essential amino acid that can initiate restful sleep. Chamomile is a good source of tryptophan and makes a delicate, tasty tea. Traditional herbal medicine has used valerian root as a sleep inducer; now this gentle herbal remedy is widely available both in Europe and the United States. Though valerian has an unpleasant taste, it is palatable in capsule form. Both valerian root and chamomile are also effective in relieving indigestion and intestinal gas. Peppermint is another soothing herb that helps to relax tense muscles and that can be taken as a tea.

Muscle-Relaxant Herbs. Several Oriental herbs have been used for thousands of years for the treatment of menstrual cramps because they have a direct relaxant effect on the uterine muscle. These herbs are available in the United States in health food stores and herbal shops. Dong quai, or *angelica root extract*, is considered an important relaxant herb in Oriental medicine. It causes an initial increase in uterine tension and contraction, which is then followed by uterine relaxation. Angelica root extract has significant pain-relieving properties as well, rivaling the effectiveness of aspirin. Peony root is often used in combination with angelica in the treatment of menstrual cramps; it has similar physiological effects on the uterine muscle, but its relaxant effect is more pronounced. Cramp bark is an American herb often used to treat menstrual cramps. It contains high doses of vitamin C and may help to relax the muscle by improving capillary permeability, which aids the flow of essential nutrients to the tense muscle and helps remove the waste products that can worsen cramping, such as lactic acid. Black cohosh, unicorn root, and black haw bark also have a long history in American herbology as effective remedies for menstrual cramps. I have used these herbs often with patients who have, subsequently, noted significant relief of menstrual discomfort.

Anti-Inflammatory Herbs. In both the Oriental and Western healing traditions, white willow has a long and distinguished history as an effective pain reliever. Its active painkilling chemical, salicin, was isolated around 1828 by French and German chemists. Years later, salicylic acid, the precursor of aspirin, was purified. Another natural source of this aspirin precursor was discovered a short time later in the herb meadow sweet. Both meadow sweet and white willow bark reduce inflammation, pain, and fever. They can be used effectively to help treat menstrual cramps and menstrual headaches since they are able to suppress the action of the series-2 prostaglandins. Unfortunately, like aspirin, they can produce the unwanted side effects of gastric indigestion, nausea, and diarrhea, so use these herbs carefully.

Blood-Circulation Enhancers. Certain herbs such as ginger and ginkgo biloba improve circulation to the pelvis and lower extremities. Ginger causes a widening or dilation of the blood vessels. Better blood circulation helps to draw nutrients to the contracted uterus and low back muscles and also helps to remove waste products like lactic acid and carbon dioxide. Ginger also has an antispasmodic effect on the smooth muscle of the intestinal tract and can help to relieve the digestive symptoms that occur with menstrual cramps, including nausea, vomiting, and bowel changes. Ginger is obviously a helpful herb for women with menstrual cramps.

Besides taking ginger in tincture or capsule form, you can also take it as a tea. To make ginger tea, buy a fresh ginger root from your local supermarket. Grate a few teaspoons of the fresh root into a quart pot of water. Bring it to a boil, then steep for 30 minutes. This is a very soothing herbal tea, delicious with a small amount of honey.

Ginkgo biloba also improves blood circulation and oxygenation to the pelvic region and lower extremities. It has a vasodilating effect and slows metabolic processes during a period of decreased blood supply. It is a very powerful herbal remedy and can be effectively combined with ginger.

CHAPTER 5

Endometriosis

*E*ndometriosis is a medical condition that occurs when the cells that comprise the lining of the uterus (or endometrium) break away and implant themselves in the pelvis. Once outside the uterine cavity, these cells can grow on many pelvic structures. They are commonly found on the ovaries, bowel, appendix, bladder, ligaments of the uterus, and cervix. They can even invade distant areas of the body, implanting on the lungs or armpit.

These implants respond to hormonal stimulation (particularly, high estrogen levels) just as the regular lining of the uterus does. As a result, these implants can bleed within the pelvic cavity on a monthly basis. However, unlike the regular uterine lining, bleeding from endometriosis-related implants cannot leave the body with the regular monthly menstrual flow. Instead, the blood remains trapped within the pelvis. Over time, it causes inflammation, scar tissue, cysts, and other structural damage to the organs and tissues in this area. In severe cases, the scar tissue formed can be so dense that it obliterates the ovaries, fallopian tubes, and other pelvic structures.

Endometriosis is actually a relatively common gynecological problem. It affects as many as five million American women (7 to 15 percent of the female population). It is found primarily in women between the ages of twenty to forty-five, with the peak incidence in women in their thirties and forties. However, even teenagers have been diagnosed with endometriosis. The problem has resurfaced, though rarely, in post-menopausal women, reactivated by the estrogen replacement therapy used for relief of menopausal symptoms.

Endometriosis can be the cause of significant pain and disability. While 30 percent of all women with endometriosis have no symptoms because the implants have lodged away from nerves and important pelvic organs, 70 percent of women with this condition experience severe and recurrent symptoms. The most common symptoms include progressively worsening menstrual cramps and pain (affecting 60 percent of women with endometriosis), pain during sexual intercourse, infertility (30 percent are unable to conceive), and premenstrual spotting and excessive menstrual flow (30 percent). Other symptoms include increased urinary frequency, pain during urination, blood in the urine during menstruation, rectal bleeding, and painful bowel movements or constipation when the implants invade the bladder or bowels. Occasionally cysts form which are deep brown in color (known as "chocolate cysts"). These cysts are filled with old blood and endometrial cells. They tend to grow fast and can even leak blood, which can be quite painful.

In severe cases of endometriosis, a combination of medical therapy and lifestyle modification may be the best course of action. Medical therapies range from surgical procedures (including hysterectomy for severe cases that have much pelvic scarring), to the use of low-dose birth control pills and medications which suppress ovulation, thereby reducing estrogenic stimulation of the implants. A variety of self-care techniques can also help to lower estrogen levels in the body. These include elimination from the diet of saturated fats from dairy and meat source, as well as avoidance of chocolate, sugar, salt, and caffeine. A high-fiber, vegetarian-based diet is optimal. Avoidance of excessive emotional stress which can affect ovulation adversely is helpful, too.

Vitamins and Minerals for Endometriosis

The following vitamins, minerals, and herbs can be helpful for women with endometriosis:

Vitamin A. Bleeding can be a problem for women with endometriosis. (One-third of patients complain of excessive flow and spotting). Fortunately, vitamin A can play a role in reducing these symptoms. In a study of 71 women with excessive bleeding, these women were found to have significantly lower blood levels of vitamin A than the normal population. Almost 90 percent of the women studied returned to a normal bleeding pattern after two weeks of vitamin A treatment.

There are two types of vitamin A. Vitamin A from animal sources is usually derived from fish liver and is oil soluble. This type of vitamin A can be toxic if taken in too large a dose (more than 25,000 IU per day, if taken longer than a few months). In contrast, beta carotene—the precursor of vitamin A found in plants—for most people, is not toxic in large amounts. The many excellent food sources of beta carotene include yellow, red, and orange fruits and vegetables such as sweet potatoes, carrot juice, apricots, papayas, and cantelopes. Dark green vegetables like broccoli and kale are also good sources.

Vitamin B Complex. Vitamin B complex helps to regulate estrogen levels by promoting efficient estrogen metabolism by the liver. The liver converts the most potent form of estrogen (estradiol) to weaker forms (estrone and estriol), which can then be disposed of by the body. Since endometriosis can be triggered by excess estrogen, it is important that estrogen levels are properly regulated by the liver. A pioneering study in 1942 and 1943, underscored the important role of several B-complex vitamins in regulating estrogen levels by promoting healthy liver function. Women with several problems related to excessive estrogen levels, including heavy menstrual flow, PMS, and fibrocystic breast disease received supplements of vitamin B complex. When supplemented with thiamine (B_1), riboflavin (B_2), niacin, and niacinamide (B_3), as well as the rest of the B complex, the women in this study showed relief of estrogen-related symptoms.

Vitamin B_6 is also an important factor in the production of the beneficial series-1 prostaglandins. Series-1 prostaglandins have a relaxant effect on uterine muscles as well as an anti-inflammatory effect on various tissues. As a result, they can help to reduce symptoms of endometriosis and, possibly, help limit the spread of implants. In addition, because vitamin B_6 levels drop in women using the birth control pill—a common treatment for both spasmodic dysmenorrhea and endometriosis—they should take supplemental B_6. They can safely take B_6 in doses up to 300 mg. They should avoid taking a dose above this level because it can be neurotoxic.

In women with endometriosis, I generally recommend 50 to 100 mg per day of vitamin B complex, with additional B_6 (up to 300 mg total daily dose), if appropriate. The B vitamins are water-soluble and easily lost from the body. In fact, emotional and nutritional stress accelerate the loss of these essential nutrients from the body and can worsen symptoms of endometriosis. Besides supplementation, a diet high in B complex is desirable for women. The B-complex vitamins are commonly found in food such as whole grains, beans and peas, and liver.

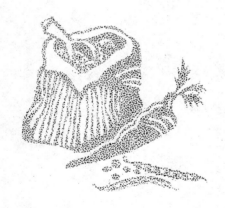

Vitamin C. Vitamin C has been tested, along with bio-flavonoids, as a treatment for heavy and irregular menstrual bleeding. One third of women with endometriosis have excessive bleeding or spotting. One project testing the effects of supplemental vitamin C showed a reduction in bleeding in 87 percent of the participants. Vitamin C helps reduce bleeding by strengthening capillaries and preventing capillary fragility. Women who do bleed excessively may eventually become iron-deficient and anemic. Vitamin C helps increase iron absorption from food sources such as bran, peas, seeds, nuts, and leafy green vegetables. This can help prevent iron deficiency anemia in women with heavy bleeding.

Vitamin C is also an important antistress vitamin essential for healthy adrenal function and immune function. The vitamin may help to limit the spread of endometrial implants by stimulating immune function and limiting inflammation and scarring. It can also help decrease the fatigue and lethargy symptoms that accompany cramps.

I recommend that women with excessive bleeding and cramps consume between 1000 to 4000 mg of vitamin C per day, especially when symptoms occur. Many fruits and vegetables are excellent sources of vitamin C.

Bioflavonoids. Like vitamin C, bioflavonoids, or vitamin P, have also shown dramatic results in their ability to reduce heavy and irregular menstrual bleeding and spotting. This occurs through two mechanisms:

1. Bioflavonoids strengthen the capillary walls. In conjunction with vitamin C, bioflavonoids have been used in women with bleeding problems due to hormonal imbalance, and have been tested in women who have lost multiple pregnancies due to bleeding.

2. Bioflavonoids are weakly estrogenic and antiestrogenic.

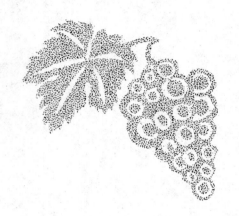

Though these plants are estrogenic, the doses found are much weaker than the levels in drugs. (Bioflavonoids contain 1/50,000 the potency of a drug dose of estrogen.) For women with endometriosis, they help regulate and reduce estrogen levels by interfering with estrogen production. Bioflavonoidal estrogen can compete with the body's estrogen precursors for space on the binding sites of enzymes. They can also compete with the estrogens manufactured by the body by binding with the estrogen receptors of the cells in such estrogen-sensitive target organs as the uterus and breast.

Thus, on one hand, bioflavonoids can act to lower estrogen levels in the body of women with fibroids and endometriosis whose symptoms are triggered by excessive estrogen. On the other hand, the weakly estrogenic effect of bioflavonoids can actually help relieve symptoms such as hot flashes, night sweats, and mood swings in menopausal women who are deficient in estrogen. As a result, bioflavonoids help to normalize estrogen levels, reducing it in women who suffer from excessive levels, and boosting it in women who are deficient.

Nature provides us with many excellent food sources of bioflavonoids. These include soybeans, buckwheat, alfalfa, the inner peel and pulp of citrus fruits, grape skins, and many brightly colored berries. Bioflavonoids are often found in fruits and vegetables that are high in vitamin C, thereby pairing a healthful combination for women with endometriosis.

Vitamin E. Like bioflavonoids, this essential nutrient has been used to relieve symptoms of diseases triggered by an imbalance in estrogen levels (and other female hormones). These include PMS, fibrocystic breast disease and breast tenderness, menstrual cramps, and menopausal symptoms. However, unlike bioflavonoids, it is not entirely clear how vitamin E causes this "smoothing out" of the hormonal effect on the body. One study, conducted in the 1980s by physicians affiliated with

Johns Hopkins University Medical School, researched this question. Their conclusion was that vitamin E does have a powerful effect on the endocrine system—but they could still not pinpoint the exact mechanism driving this phenomenon.

I have found vitamin E to be a useful part of a treatment program for the relief of endometriosis (and the relief of other accompanying problems such as PMS and fibrocystic breast disease). The best natural sources of vitamin E are wheat germ oil, walnut oil, soybean oil, and other grain and seed oil sources. I generally recommend that women with endometriosis consume between 400 to 2000 IU per day. Women with hypertension and diabetes should start on a much lower dose of vitamin E (100 IU per day). Any increase in dosage should be made slowly and monitored carefully. Otherwise, vitamin E tends to be extremely safe and is taken by millions of people.

Essential Fatty Acids. Sufficient essential fatty acids are an extremely important part of the nutritional program for any woman with menstrual cramps, whether or not they are due to endometriosis. The prostaglandins made from essential fatty acids have muscle-relaxant and blood vessel-relaxant properties that can significantly reduce muscle cramps and tension. They also have an anti-inflammatory effect on tissues, which is very important in limiting inflammation within the endometrial implants, and thereby painful pelvic symptoms.

The essential fatty acids, linoleic acid, and linolenic acid, are derived from specific food sources in our diet—primarily raw seeds and nuts and certain fish like salmon, mackerel, and trout. Unlike other fats, such as the unhealthy saturated fats, these fats cannot be made by the body and must be supplied daily in our diets, either from food or supplements.

To efficiently convert fatty acids to prostaglandins, a number of other nutrients must be present. For example, the conversion of linoleic acid to GLA (leading to the creation of the beneficial series-1 prostaglandins) requires the presence of magnesium, zinc, vitamin B_6, vitamin C, and niacin. Women who are deficient in these nutrients can't make the chemical conversions effectively. In addition, diet is a factor with women who consume a great deal of cholesterol, processed oils, and alcohol. Other factors that impede prostaglandin production include emotional stress, diabetes, allergies, and eczema. In women with these risk factors, less than 1 percent of linoleic acid might be converted to GLA.

Anti-Inflammatory Herbs. Several anti-inflammatory herbs may help relieve symptoms of endometriosis and reduce inflammation of implants. White willow bark is an effective pain reliever containing salicin, an active pain-killing chemical. The precursor of aspirin, salicylic acid, was purified from this plant. Another natural source of this aspirin precursor is meadow sweet. Both meadow sweet and white willow bark reduce inflammation, pain, and fever. They help treat primary menstrual cramps, menstrual headaches, and the pain symptoms of endometriosis because they suppress the action of F_2 Alpha prostaglandins. They can, however, produce the unwanted side effects of gastric indigestion, nausea, and diarrhea, so these herbs should be used carefully.

Phytoestrogens. Other herbs besides bioflavonoids are weakly estrogenic. These include anise, fennel, licorice, black cohosh, blessed thistle, false unicorn root, and a host of other plants. Like bioflavonoids, these herbs have a hormone-balancing effect and help lower excessive estrogen levels and control heavy bleeding symptoms or spotting. The potency of phytoestrogens varies between 1/400 to 1/50,000 of that of synthetic estrogen or estradiol, the main type of estrogen made by the ovaries during a woman's active reproductive years.

CHAPTER 6

Fibrocystic Breast Disease

Thirty percent of American women have fibrocystic breast disease, a benign (noncancerous) condition characterized by round lumps that move freely within the breast tissue. This lumps are usually tender to the touch. In contrast, a cancerous growth in the breast is often not tender or freely movable when touched. The texture of the lumps can vary from soft to firm. For many women, the tenderness may increase as menstruation approaches. Often the cysts fill with fluid and can enlarge premenstrually in response to the increase in hormonal levels during this time.

The main hormones implicated in the worsening of breast symptoms premenstrually include estrogen, the main female hormone, and prolactin, the milk-release hormone secreted by the pituitary gland. Dietary factors have also been implicated. These include caffeine intake from coffee, black teas, colas, and chocolate, as well as excessive saturated fat and salt. Usually the symptoms of pain and swelling do not persist once menstruation begins, and most women notice significant relief at this time. The difference in the breast swelling can be so marked between the first and second half of the menstrual cycle that some women actually change bra size.

With repeated cycles of hormonal stimulation, the breast cysts may become chronically inflamed and surrounded by fibrous tissue which can harden and thicken the cysts. It is then more difficult for the fluid trapped in the cysts to escape and be reabsorbed by the body. This condition occurs most frequently in women in their late thirties and forties. To distinguish these hardened cysts from cancer, physicians often perform a simple office procedure called a needle aspiration. In this procedure, a needle is used to remove fluid from the cyst. This helps relieve pressure from the cyst on the surrounding tissue if it is causing pain, as well as rule out breast cancer. A mammogram will also help distinguish a breast cyst from breast cancer.

However, if there is a lingering concern about making an accurate diagnosis, a surgical biopsy might be performed. This is done under a local anesthetic in a physician's office or clinic or under general anesthesia in a hospital setting. A biopsy allows the physician to remove the entire breast mass so that the cells can be examined microscopically for any cancerous changes. Fortunately, most masses are benign.

Besides eliminating certain foods from the diet (caffeine, saturated fats, and salt), a high-fiber diet, including many plant-based foods, fruits and vegetables, beans and peas, raw seeds and nuts, and whole grains may help prevent cyclical fluctuations in cyst size and tenderness. The addition of seafood to the diet, particularly fish, may be useful in preventing breast cysts due to the iodine content and healthy oils contained in certain fish. The best fish for female health include those high in the Omega-3 fatty acids like salmon, trout, and mackerel.

Vitamins and Minerals for Breast Cysts

The following vitamins and minerals can be helpful in reducing and preventing breast cysts:

Vitamin A. Vitamin A has been found to be useful in reducing both the pain symptoms and the size of the breast lesions in women with fibrocystic breast disease. At the University of Montreal Medical School, where high doses of vitamin A were administered (150,000 IU daily) to a small research group of volunteer women. The women studied had documented benign breast disease with moderate to severe pain symptoms. Their breast tenderness had not previously responded to mild analgesic medication (painkillers) or cessation of caffeine use. Eighty percent of the women tested had beneficial results with vitamin A and a dramatic reduction in the level of pain. The lessening of breast pain was still evident eight months after the study ended. Forty percent of the women had at least a 50 percent decrease in the size of their breast lumps. One drawback, though, is that vitamin A in high doses can cause toxic symptoms. Vitamin A derived from fish sources is an oil-based product which can accumulate to high levels in the liver, where it is stored. Several women in this study had severe headaches from the high dosage of vitamin A taken, and several other women had more mild side effects.

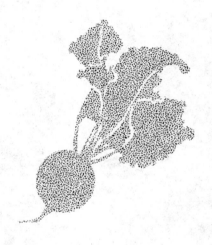

To avoid the risk of side effects from fish oil-based vitamin A, it is safer for most women to use the provitamin A, beta carotene. Beta carotene is found abundantly in many yellow, orange, red, and dark green fruits and vegetables. It is converted to vitamin A by the liver and intestines as needed by the body. In fact, many women who eat a plant-based diet can easily ingest 50,000 to 100,000 IU of beta carotene on a daily basis. (One cup of carrot juice or one sweet potato contains 20,000

IU of beta carotene). Supplements of beta carotene are also readily available in health food stores and pharmacies.

Vitamin E. In several controlled studies, vitamin E was found to be quite helpful in reducing the pain and tenderness, as well as the size, of breast lumps. In one study, where subjects were given 600 IU of vitamin E for two menstrual cycles, 80 percent showed a positive response. Another study of 29 women with fibrocystic breast lumps, which worsen premenstrually, showed again a good response to vitamin E treatments. At doses of 500 or 600 IU per day, 16 women had moderate to total symptom relief. The other 13 women had reduction of cyst size or complete disappearance of the cysts.

Iodine. In animal studies, iodine-deficient rats were found to develop breast changes similar to human fibrocystic disease. Human studies have also suggested that women who are iodine deficient may have a predisposition towards developing breast cysts. Iodine is needed by the body for the production of the thyroid hormone. Lack of adequate thyroid hormone also affects the menstrual cycle.

Sea vegetables such as nori, kelp, and dulse, found in the produce section of health food stores, are good sources of iodine. Dulse is also available in liquid drops, while kelp is available in tablets. Kelp also comes in powdered form and can be used in cooking as a good salt substitute.

Essential Fatty Acids. Several studies have looked at the beneficial effects of evening primrose oil on fibrocystic breast disease. Evening primrose oil is an excellent source of the essential fatty acid, linoleic acid, and its chemical derivative, gamma linolenic acid (GLA). In one study of 291 women with severe breast pain, 45 percent of the women had symptom relief with the use of evening primrose oil. Another study of 41 women showed equally good symptom relief. The beneficial results were maintained in women who continued to use evening primrose oil after the study ended. Typical dosages used were 1500 mg twice a day. (This would amount to taking 6 of the 500 mg capsules commonly available.) In my experience, some women need to go as high as 9 to 12 capsules per day for relief of severe symptoms. Borage oil and black currant oil are more concentrated sources of GLA, so the number of capsules necessary is reduced. For example, 3 or 4 capsules per day of borage oil may be sufficient.

CHAPTER 7

Anemia, Heavy Menstrual Flow, and Irregularity

Anemia

Anemia is characterized by a reduction in the number of red blood cells in the body or a reduction in hemoglobin (the oxygen-carrying protein in red blood cells). Anemia reduces the amount of oxygen available to all cells of the body; thus, carbon dioxide, a waste product, accumulates in the cells and cannot be removed by the lungs with normal breathing. As a result of the blood's lower oxygen-carrying capability, the cells for the body's normal chemical functioning have less available energy. Important processes, such as muscular activity and cell building and repair, slow down and become less efficient. More than 95 percent of the body's chemical reactions depend upon optimal oxygen levels in cells and tissues.

As a result, the symptoms of anemia can be very debilitating, affecting many organ systems of the body. Usual signs of anemia are fatigue, dizziness, general weakness, paleness, loss of appetite, brittle and ridged nails, abdominal pain, sore tongue, yellowing of the skin, tingling in the hands and feet, loss of coordination, and diarrhea.

Anemia is a very common health problem, affecting as many as 20 percent of all American women. Yet it is often overlooked or misdiagnosed since its symptoms are similar to those of many other problems. Your health care practitioner can easily tell whether or not you're anemic by a simple blood test. When evaluating the blood sample for anemia, the total number of red blood cells are counted. The percentage of blood that is made up of red blood cells, or the hematocrit, is estimated by determining the ratio of red blood cells to the whole blood. In healthy women, the hematocrit averages 38 to 47 percent; it is lower in women with anemia. The hemoglobin is also estimated because it is reduced in people with anemia. For healthy women, normal hemoglobin ranges between 12 to 15 grams per deciliter. If you are anemic, further blood testing can determine the specific nutritional deficiencies that cause the problem.

The most common forms of anemia are caused by the lack of essential nutrients needed for normal blood cell production—iron, folic acid, and vitamin B_{12}. Other nutritional deficiencies, such as a lack of vitamin B_6, vitamin A, vitamin E, copper, and zinc, can also increase the risk of developing anemia.

Iron-deficiency anemia is the most common type of anemia. When women are iron-deficient, their red blood cells do not mature properly; instead, they remain small and pale-colored. The reason for these low iron reserves? Women simply don't eat enough iron-rich foods or take iron supplements. Many women diet excessively, so their caloric intake does not contain sufficient foods to sustain an adequate iron reserve. For some women, dairy products such as yogurt, cheese, and cottage cheese constitute their main source of protein. Not only are dairy products very low in iron, but research has shown that excessive dairy products in the diet actually impedes the absorption of iron from other sources. Women, especially teenagers, who constantly eat junk food like candy bars or potato chips, are also at high risk.

One of the most common ways women become iron-deficient is through blood loss during their periods (even more iron can be lost in women with heavy menstrual periods). Because iron is lost monthly, it must be replaced—if not, the risk of iron-deficiency anemia increases. Pregnancy is another time of iron loss; a woman's blood increases in volume to support the fetus. Iron is very important in forming the baby's blood and supplying oxygen to the baby's cells and tissues. Iron is also lost through the breast milk of nursing mothers because this important mineral is used to fortify the newborn infant.

Other women with low iron stores include those with celiac disease (gluten intolerance), frequent aspirin users (because of the slight internal bleeding aspirin can cause), IUD wearers (because of the heavy menstrual flow), and those who donate more than two pints of blood per year. Your goal is to minimize this excessive blood loss, and with it, the loss of iron stores.

To maintain your iron stores and prevent iron-deficiency anemia, it is necessary to take adequate iron on a daily basis, either in food or supplemental form. Good sources include millet, wheat germ, pinto beans, garbanzo beans, kidney beans, broccoli, brussels sprouts, greens, sweet potatoes, Swiss chard, prune juice, figs, and raisins. Flax seeds (the raw seeds ground into a powder, not the oil) are very high in iron. For the most efficient use of this iron, combine the foods mentioned above with fruits high in vitamin C: oranges, dates, blackberries, pineapple, cherries, bilberries, seeds such as sesame and sunflower, tahini, and peas. Food sources of the other most common causes of anemia (folic acid and B_{12}-deficiencies) include: spinach, kale, and Swiss chard for folic acid, and meat and eggs (or supplemental forms for vegetarian women) for vitamin B_{12}.

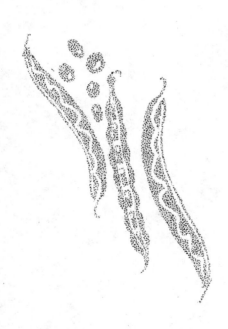

Heavy Menstrual Flow and Irregularity

At either end of the reproductive cycle, in puberty or during perimenopause (the time of transition into menopause), women often experience irregular periods or heavy menstrual flow. During adolescence, a woman's estrogen levels are gradually increasing. While her menstrual cycle is in the process of establishing itself on a mature adult basis, ovulation is often infrequent or sporadic. As a result, an adolescent may have periods that are heavier, longer, or closer together than those of adult women. Menstrual cycles that occur without ovulation are called anovulatory cycles. After a few years of menstruation, this pattern of heavy menstrual bleeding tends to self-correct as ovulation begins to occur on a regular basis.

At the other end of the spectrum, as women approach menopause, their follicles gradually atrophy and diminish in number. This transition period can last as long as four to five years. As their follicles lose the ability to produce estrogen and progesterone, perimenopausal women begin to ovulate less frequently.

For many women, the transitions into menopause can be uncomfortable and difficult. As the hormonal output becomes unstable during a woman's mid to late forties, irregular heavy bleeding can occur. The menstrual cycle often shortens, with periods coming closer together. Bleeding can become heavier and last longer. A one-week to ten-day menstrual period is fairly common. Some patients tell me that their cycles are unpredictable, with periods sometimes occurring twice a month, and, in some extreme cases, lasting as long as 60 or more days. This blood loss can be dangerous because it can lead to anemia if not treated. Luckily, this problem tends to self-correct. When menopause approaches, the periods occur at longer intervals and the flow becomes light and scanty until menstruation finally ceases.

During a phase of heavy menstrual bleeding, some women are likely to need medical care. Often the bleeding can be stopped by a synthetic progesteronelike hormone called progestin. Provera is the type that is used most often in the United States. Provera is taken orally for one or two weeks and usually stops the bleeding. It acts in much the same way as natural progesterone, limiting the amount of bleeding from the uterine lining during the second half of the menstrual cycle.

For some women, the use of progestins is not sufficient, and an operation called a dilatation and curettage (D&C) must be performed. The D&C effectively stops the bleeding by removing the lining of the uterus through a scraping or suction technique while the patient is under anesthesia. The D&C is useful in ruling out other potentially more serious causes of bleeding. After the D&C, cells of the uterine lining are analyzed for abnormalities such as uterine polyps or cancer. In extreme cases, when the bleeding cannot be easily controlled, a hysterectomy, or removal of the uterus, is performed.

Lifestyle modification can play a major role in regulating menstrual periods. In fact, healthier lifestyle habits can often help reduce bleeding and the likelihood that a woman will need a hysterectomy. Women bleed more during times of emotional upset since stress affects hormonal levels in the body. Thus, attention to managing stress effectively is mandatory in women with heavy menstrual bleeding and irregularity. A diet high in saturated fat, sugar, and alcohol can increase estrogen levels and cause excessive build-up of cells in the uterine lining. Obesity is also a risk factor for heavy menstrual bleeding. For regulation of menstrual cycles, a low-fat, low-sugar diet is necessary. An optimal diet contains plenty of high-nutrient foods, such as whole grains, beans, peas, fresh fruits and vegetables, raw seeds and nuts, and fish (for women who eat meat as the main source of protein). Women who eat a nutrient-poor diet are also at high risk of heavy menstrual bleeding because they lack the nutrients to regulate normal blood flow. Medical studies have shown that deficiencies of vitamin A, vitamin C, iron, and bioflavonoids can worsen or even cause heavy, irregular menstrual bleeding.

Vitamins and Minerals for Anemia, Heavy Menstrual Bleeding, and Irregularity

Following are important nutrients for these problems:

Vitamin A. Vitamin A is needed for the healthy production of red blood cells. A study of middle-aged men on a diet deficient in vitamin A was found that the subjects' hemoglobin count started to decline even before a change in night vision or a measurable deficiency in vitamin A levels was noted. Similarly, vitamin A also plays a significant role in the prevention of heavy menstrual bleeding. In a study of 71 women with excessive menstrual bleeding, the test subjects were found to have significantly lower blood levels of vitamin A than the normal population. Almost 90 percent of the women studied returned to a normal bleeding pattern after two weeks of vitamin A treatment.

Vitamin A from animal sources usually is derived from fish liver and is oil soluble. This type of vitamin A can be toxic if taken in too large a dose (more than 25,000 IU per day, if taken longer than a few months). In contrast, beta carotene, the precursor of vitamin A found in plants, is water soluble and is not toxic in large amounts.

Vitamin B Complex. Many of the B-complex vitamins are also necessary for the prevention and reversal of anemia. A deficiency of vitamin B_1 (thiamine), vitamin B_2 (riboflavin), vitamin

B_5 (pantothenic acid), and vitamin B_6 (pyridoxine) may cause anemia, even in people who have no deficiencies in iron, folic acid, or vitamin B_{12}. The B-complex vitamins are commonly found in foods such as whole grains, beans and peas, and liver. These vitamins are water soluble. When a woman experiences emotional stress, the B-complex vitamins are more easily lost from the body. This can worsen the fatigue and lack of vitality from which women with anemia and heavy menstrual bleeding already suffer.

Folic Acid. Folic acid is one of the B-complex vitamins and plays an important role in the production of red blood cells. A deficiency of folic acid leads to anemia that cannot be corrected by supplemental iron. With folic acid deficiency, red blood cells do not mature properly; they are large and irregularly shaped. Drugs that interfere with proper absorption of folic acid include sulfa drugs and other antibiotics, phenobarbital, alcohol, and anticonvulsants used in the treatment of epilepsy. Women with folic acid-deficiency anemia are prone to symptoms such as sore tongue, digestive disturbances, forgetfulness, and mental confusion. Food sources of folic acid include oysters, salmon, whole grains, and green leafy vegetables.

Vitamin B_{12}. Vitamin B_{12} is a water-soluble vitamin that plays an important role in the production of red blood cells. Like folic acid deficiency, a B_{12} deficiency causes retardation in the growth and development of the red blood cells. B_{12}-deficient cells are immature and can develop only to a certain point. As with folic acid deficiency, these cells are large and abnormally shaped. Vitamin B_{12} is poorly absorbed from the gastrointestinal tract if the intrinsic factor, a necessary enzyme, is deficient. Because vitamin B_{12} is found primarily in meat, vegetarians may be at risk of developing a B_{12} deficiency.

Symptoms of this deficiency develop slowly and may not become apparent for as long as five or six years after the body's supply of B_{12} has been restricted. A lack of B_{12} causes brain and nervous system damage. Symptoms include shooting pains, pins-and-needles or hot-and-cold sensations in the extremities, as well as numbness, stiffness, and difficulty in walking. This deficiency can also cause mental disturbances similar to psychosis, memory defects, and mental slowness. In order to treat B_{12}-deficiency anemia (also known as pernicious anemia), the digestive tract must be bypassed and the B_{12} given as injections. Vegans (vegetarians eating no milk or egg products) should take oral supplements of B_{12} on a daily basis in small amounts.

Vitamin C. Vitamin C markedly increases iron absorption from the nonheme or vegetarian iron sources such as bran, peas, seeds, nuts, and leafy green vegetables. This can help to prevent iron deficiency anemia. Vitamin C has also been tested, along with bioflavonoids, as a treatment for heavy menstrual bleeding. One study showed a reduction in bleeding in 87 percent of the subjects. Vitamin C helps to strengthen capillaries and prevent the capillary fragility that can lead to excessive bleeding. Many fruits and vegetables are excellent sources of vitamin C.

Bioflavonoids. This is one of the most important nutrients for women at midlife. Bioflavonoids have chemical activity similar to estrogen, but have a much weaker potency than drug levels of estrogen. As a result, bioflavonoids can be used as an estrogen substitute to help regulate estrogen levels in the body. High estrogen levels are common cause of heavy menstrual bleeding and menstrual irregularity. Bioflavonoids compete with the body's production of estrogen and help to lower estrogen levels, which can limit menstrual flow.

Bioflavonoids have also shown dramatic results in their ability to reduce heavy menstrual bleeding by strengthening the capillary walls. In studies, both women with bleeding due to hormonal imbalance and women who have lost multiple pregnancies due to bleeding responded positively to bioflavonoids combined with vitamin C. Bioflavonoids can be found naturally with vitamin C in many fruits and vegetables such as grape skins, cherries, blackberries, and blueberries. Bioflavonoids are also abundant in citrus fruits, especially in the pulp and the white rind. Other excellent food sources include buckwheat and soy products.

Vitamin E. Vitamin E can act as an estrogen substitute. Like bioflavonoids, it has been studied as a treatment for various estrogen-related problems like PMS, fibrocystic breast disease, and menopause. I have found it helpful for women with menstrual flow problems and irregularity. Unlike bioflavonoids, it is not yet known precisely how vitamin E's effect on the hormones actually works.

Vitamin E is also an important antioxidant. It protects the cells from the destructive effects of environmental pollutants that can react with the cell membrane. It has been found to increase red blood cell survival and, for this reason, is an important nutrient for the prevention of anemia. Vitamin E is found abundantly in wheat germ, nuts, seeds, and some fruits and vegetables.

Iron. Women who suffer from heavy menstrual bleeding tend to be iron-deficient. In fact, some studies have found that inadequate iron intake may be a cause of excessive bleeding as well as an effect of the problem. Women who suffer from heavy menstrual bleeding should have their red blood count checked to see if supplemental iron is necessary, in addition to adopting a high-iron diet.

Heme iron, the iron from meat sources such as liver, is much better absorbed and assimilated than nonheme iron, the iron from vegetarian sources. To be absorbed properly, nonheme iron must be taken with at least 75 mg of vitamin C.

Iron deficiency is the main cause of anemia. Iron is an essential component of red blood cells, combining with protein and copper to make hemoglobin, the pigment of the red blood cells. Iron deficiency is common during all phases of a woman's life and is a frequent cause of fatigue and low-energy states. Food sources of iron include liver, blackstrap molasses, beans and peas, seeds and nuts, and certain fruits and vegetables.

Copper. Copper aids in the formation of red blood cells. A deficiency of copper is associated with anemia, as copper is necessary for proper iron absorption. Copper is found in all body tissues and is present in many of the enzymes that break down and build up body tissues. The best food sources of copper include liver, whole grains, legumes, seafood, and green leafy vegetables.

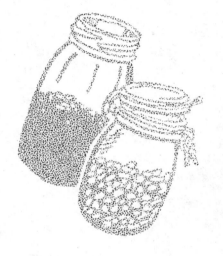

Zinc. Zinc plays an important role in the body. It is a constituent of many enzymes involved both in metabolism and digestion. It is also needed for the proper growth and development of female reproductive organs and for the normal functioning of the male prostate gland. Food sources of zinc include wheat germ, pumpkin seeds, whole grains, wheat bran, and high-protein foods. People with sickle-cell anemia may be deficient in zinc. One interesting study showed a decrease in the number of sickled red blood cells in patients who used zinc supplementation.

Herbs for Anemia, Heavy Menstrual Bleeding, and Irregularity

Herbs That Regulate Blood Loss

Two herbs have been traditionally used to stop excessive menstrual flow and postpartum hemorrhage: goldenseal and shepherd's purse. Recent research has supported the traditional claims made for these herbs. Goldenseal contains berberine, a chemical that calms uterine muscular tension. It has also been used to calm and soothe the digestive tract. Shepherd's purse helps promote blood clotting and has also been used to help stop menstrual bleeding. If your bleeding is excessive or irregular, consult your physician. This needs to be evaluated carefully by your physician who, if necessary, should institute medical therapy. Excessive and irregular bleeding can be dangerous and should never be allowed to continue without medical help. For those women for whom the menstrual flow is normal but somewhat heavier than usual, the mild properties of herbs may be helpful for symptom relief.

Plants that contain bioflavonoids may also help stop and prevent heavy menstrual bleeding. Bioflavonoids help to strengthen capillaries and reduce capillary fragility, and, along with vitamin C, can help prevent excessive bruising as well as bleeding. Bioflavonoids are found in a wide variety of fruits and flowers and are responsible for their striking colors. Good sources of bioflavonoids include citrus fruits, bilberries, cherries, and grape skins. Bioflavonoids have also been found in red clover and in some clover strains in Australia.

Many studies have demonstrated the usefulness of citrus bioflavonoids in treating a variety of bleeding problems in addition to those related to menopause, including habitual spontaneous abortion and tuberculosis. The wild yam root has been found to have the hormonal properties of progesterone. It has been used like progesterone or progestin to help regulate heavier menstrual bleeding found in women who are in transition into menopause.

Herbs Containing Iron

Other herbs help prevent anemia by providing good sources of nonheme iron. Excellent examples are yellow dock and pau d'arco. Yellow dock is also used to help promote liver health—an important factor in decreasing heavy bleeding through regulation of excessive estrogen levels, since the liver breaks down estrogen and prepares it for excretion from the body. Turmeric, or curcumin, is also used to promote liver health in traditional medicine. Recent research suggests that it has antibacterial properties. Turmeric is a delicious herb used for flavoring in traditional Indian dishes. Silymarin, or milk thistle, protects liver function by its flavonoid content. Flavonoids are strong antioxidants and help protect the liver from damage.

CHAPTER 8

Fibroid Tumors

The word "fibroid" is actually a misnomer, since it implies that these tumors arise from fibrous tissue. The correct medical term used by gynecologists for these growths is *leiomyoma* or *myomas* since these tumors arise from the smooth muscle layer of the uterus (also called the *myometrium*). This muscle layer lies under the inner lining of the uterus or *endometrium* which bleeds each month and causes women to have a menstrual period.

Fibroid tumors are very common, affecting at least 40 percent of all American women by the time they reach forty years of age. The tumors occur primarily in women in their twenties throughout their late forties and can sometimes extend throughout menopause, affecting women in their fifties and older.

Fibroids are benign growths that can arise in muscle tissue anywhere in the body but are found most commonly in the uterus. Unlike cancer, they do not invade surrounding tissue or distant organs and prove fatal if untreated. In fact, less than one-half of 1 percent of fibroids ever become cancerous; and this usually occurs in postmenopausal women. Instead, these benign muscular tumors tend to remain within the confines of the uterine tissue. However, as they grow larger, they can extend their range and put pressure on neighboring organs and tissues.

Fibroids can vary in number and size. Often multiple fibroids arise over time. Physicians performing surgery on fibroids have found as many as several hundred tumors on a single woman. Fibroids range in size from tiny pinpoint areas of tissue to rare cases of tumors weighing up to 25 or more pounds.

Significant growth of the fibroids usually causes the entire uterus to enlarge. Often a gynecologist feels a firm, irregularly enlarged uterus with smoothly rounded protrusions arising from the uterine wall. Gynecologists tend to describe fibroids in terms of the uterine enlargement caused by pregnancy. A woman with fibroids might be described by her physician as having a "12- to 14- week-size uterus" or even a "20- to 24- week-size uterus," which approximates a six-month pregnancy in a woman with a very large uterus.

Interestingly, not all large fibroids cause symptoms. If the fibroids grow in a way that do not put pressure on neighboring organs, a woman can live with large fibroids for many years without needing medical care. However, 50 percent of fibroids do grow in such a way as to cause symptoms, often necessitating medical care. Since these tumors are hormone-sensitive, they often grow larger and cause symptoms during periods when estrogen levels are elevated. This commonly occurs for women in their late thirties and throughout their forties as they transition into menopause. During this time, hormone levels tend to fluctuate greatly. Estrogen levels may be elevated or normal often without the gross limiting effects of the second female hormone, progesterone, which is often absent or inadequate in menopausal women. This can result in estrogenic stimulation to the uterus. Fibroids, however, can also be seen in women in their early thirties, or less commonly, in women in their twenties when other risk factors are present. These risk factors include obesity; excessive emotional stress; and a diet high in saturated fat, sugar, and alcohol, which can increase estrogen levels in the body. Conversely, a high-fiber, low-fat vegetarian-based diet is protective since it lowers estrogen levels in the body.

Symptoms of Fibroid Tumors

Bleeding. Approximately one-third of women with fibroids suffer from abnormal uterine bleeding. Many women develop a heavier menstrual flow that often lasts longer than normal. Some women develop irregular bleeding between periods. In my practice, I have seen women with fibroids develop such heavy bleeding that they actually become anemic. If not treated rapidly, this can cause significant health problems such as weakness, tiredness, and shortness of breath on exertion. If the bleeding continues unchecked, a woman can eventually require hospitalization and a surgical procedure to stop the problem. Check with your physician if you notice changes in your bleeding pattern. It is important that any significant changes in menstrual flow be evaluated as it could be due to rapidly growing fibroids or even another medical problem.

The most common cause of abnormal bleeding is submucosal fibroids. These submucosal fibroids grow into the uterine cavity and affect the lining of the uterus, or the endometrium. Intramural fibroids, which can grow into the wall of the uterus, can worsen bleeding too.

Pain. Many women with fibroids experience symptoms of pressure and pain. This may be a sense of progressive pelvic fullness or a dragging sensation. This is usually due to slowly enlarging intramural fibroids growing within the wall of the uterus or subsurosal fibroids growing on the outside of the uterus into the pelvic cavity. Such fibroids are often easy to feel on a pelvic or abdominal exam. In fact, my patients with very large fibroids are often astonished to realize that they can easily feel their own fibroids by touching their abdomens.

Fibroids that grow to the point of putting pressure on other pelvic structures may affect both the bladder and bowel functions. When pressing against the bladder, a fibroid tumor can cause a reduction in bladder capacity resulting in frequent urination and urgency. Occasionally, pressure on the ureters (the tube that brings urine from the kidney to the bladder) may lead to kidney damage. Fibroids that press on the bowels may cause constipation or hemorrhoids.

Infertility. Fibroids may be the cause of as much as 5 to 10 percent of infertility cases. There are several reasons why this is the case. Fibroids may inhibit implantation of the fertilized egg in the uterine lining by altering transport of the sperm, compressing the fallopian tube, or disrupting the lining of the uterus. In addition, fibroids may cause spontaneous abortion during the first three months of pregnancy. It is possible that this loss occurs because the fibroids distort the uterine cavity or alter blood flow that would normally be needed to nourish the growing fetus. In any case, women with a history of infertility who wish to conceive should be carefully evaluated as to the size and location of any preexisting fibroid.

Besides reducing stress and improving diet, women should take nutritional supplements to control fibroid tumors or to shrink them. (However, they do tend to shrink normally after menopause when estrogen levels are diminished.)

Vitamins and Minerals for Women with Fibroids

The following vitamins and minerals play important roles in the symptom relief and prevention of fibroids:

Vitamin A. Heavy menstrual bleeding is a significant problem for women with fibroids and is the most common reason for hysterectomies. Vitamin A can help reduce these symptoms.

Vitamin A from animal sources (usually from fish liver) is oil soluble and can be toxic if taken in overly large doses (more than 25,000 IU per day, for longer than a few months). In contrast, beta carotene, the precursor of vitamin A found in plants, is water soluble and is not toxic for most people in large amounts. Many of my patients ingest 50,000 to 100,000 IU of beta carotene daily from dietary sources.

Vitamin B Complex. Vitamin B complex promotes efficient estrogen metabolism by the liver, which helps to regulate estrogen levels in the body. It is important that estrogen levels are properly regulated through liver metabolism because fibroids can be triggered by excess estrogen in the body. Research shows that women with several problems related to excessive estrogen levels—including heavy menstrual flow, PMS, and fibrocystic breast disease—improved with supplements of vitamin B complex. In studies where women received supplements of thiamine (B_1), riboflavin (B_2), niacin, and niacinamide (B_3), and the rest of the B complex, the subjects showed relief of estrogen-related symptoms.

For women with fibroids, I generally recommend 50 to 100 mg per day of vitamin B complex, with additional B_6 (up to 300 mg total daily dose), if appropriate. The B vitamins are water soluble and easily lost from the body. Emotional and nutritional stress accelerate the body's loss of these essential nutrients and can worsen symptoms of endometriosis. Even with supplementation, a diet high in B complex is desirable for women. The B-complex vitamins are commonly found in food such as whole grains, beans and peas, and liver.

Vitamin C. Vitamin C has been tested, along with bioflavonoids, as a treatment for heavy and irregular menstrual bleeding indicative of women with fibroids. Vitamin C helps reduce bleeding by strengthening capillaries and preventing capillary fragility. Women who do bleed excessively may become iron-deficient and, eventually, anemic. Vitamin C helps increase iron absorption from food sources such as bran, peas, seeds, nuts, and leafy green vegetables. This can help prevent iron-deficiency anemia in women with heavy bleeding. I recommend that women with excessive bleeding and cramps use 1000 to 4000 mg of vitamin C per day, especially when symptoms occur. Many fruits and vegetables are excellent sources of vitamin C.

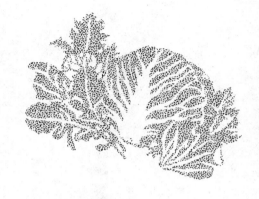

Bioflavonoids. Bioflavonoids, or vitamin P, have also shown dramatic results in their ability to reduce heavy and irregular menstrual bleeding. This occurs through two mechanisms. First, bioflavonoids strengthen the capillary walls. In conjunction with vitamin C, bioflavonoids have been used to treat women with bleeding problems due to hormonal imbalance, and have helped women who have lost multiple pregnancies due to bleeding. Second, bioflavonoids are weakly estrogenic, though the levels are much weaker than those produced by the body or found in drugs. (Bioflavonoids contain 1/50,000 of the potency of an estrogen drug.) Bioflavonoids help to regulate and reduce estrogen levels by interfering with estrogen production. They do this by binding to an enzyme called estrogen synthetase, taking over the binding sites normally occupied by male hormones. Our bodies convert male hormones to estrogen as a critical step in estrogen production. They also compete with the body's estrogens by binding with the estrogen receptors in such estrogen-sensitive target organs as the walls of the uterus and breast.

Vitamin E. Like bioflavonoids, this essential nutrient helps relieve symptoms of diseases triggered by an imbalance in estrogen levels (and other female hormones) including PMS, fibrocystic breast disease and breast tenderness, menstrual cramps, and menopausal symptoms. However, unlike bioflavonoids, it is not entirely clear how vitamin E causes this "smoothing out" of the hormonal effects on the body.

I use vitamin E as part of a therapeutic program for the relief of fibroids (and other accompanying problems such as PMS and fibrocystic breast disease.) The best natural sources of vitamin E are wheat germ oil, walnut oil, soybean oil, and other grain and seed oil sources. I generally recommend that women with fibroids take between 400 to 2000 IU per day. Women with hypertension and diabetes should start on a much lower dose of vitamin E (100 IU per day), slowly increase dosage, if needed, and monitor it carefully. Vitamin E is generally extremely safe and is taken by millions of people.

Essential Fatty Acids. Flax seed is one of the best natural sources of linoleic acid and linolenic acid. Almost 80 percent of flax oil is composed of these two essential fatty acids.

In a 1990 study reported in the *British Medical Journal,* the estrogenic properties of flax oil were tested along with soy flour in postmenopausal women. Researchers found that like other plant sources of estrogen, flax oil is considerably weaker in potency than the estrogen made by the body, and as a result, can help regulate estrogen levels downward. This can be very beneficial for women with fibroid tumors and other problems due to excessive levels of estrogen.

Flax oil can be taken as a supplement or added to food before serving. This golden oil is delicious on potatoes, rice, steamed vegetables, or toast as a butter substitute. Do not cook with flax oil, as it is heat-sensitive; it must be kept covered and refrigerated.

Ground flax meal is even better than flax oil in controlling the symptoms or growth of fibroid tumors. This is because the whole ground flax seed contains two sources of estrogen: the oil and plant lignan (the cellulose-like supportive structure of the seed). The plant lignan is not only weakly estrogenic but antiestrogenic as well. For an "anti-fibroid" cereal, combine ground flax meal with soy milk. More cereal recipes begin on page 237.

Herbs for Fibroid Tumors

Phytoestrogens. Purified bioflavonoids are available in capsule and tablet form, and they are also found in a wide variety of fruits and flowers and are responsible for the striking colors of many plants. Good sources of bioflavonoids include citrus fruits, hawthorn berries, bilberries, cherries, and grape skins. Bioflavonoids have also been found in red clover and in some clover strains in Australia. Many of these plants are available as herbal tinctures (liquid) or in capsules.

Other phytoestrogens include fennel, licorice, anise, black cohosh, blessed thistle, and false unicorn root. These herbs are also available in capsule form or as tinctures. Wild yam, an herbal source of progesterone—the other female hormone—may also be helpful in balancing and regulating hormones.

Blood Flow Regulators. Heavy menstrual bleeding is the main complaint of women with fibroid tumors. Certain herbs help stop excessive menstrual bleeding.

Women traditionally take goldenseal and shepherd's purse which recent research has proven effective in regulating menstrual flow. Goldenseal contains berberine, which calms uterine muscular tension and the digestive tract. Shepherd's purse promotes blood clotting and helps stop menstrual bleeding.

However, if your bleeding is excessive or irregular, consult your physician. Excessive and irregular bleeding can be dangerous and needs medical attention. The mild properties of these herbs relieve symptoms only in those women whose menstrual flow is close to normal but somewhat heavier than usual.

Herbal Sources of Iron. Herbal sources of nonheme iron like yellow dock and pau d'arco may be helpful for women who are anemic. Yellow dock promotes liver health—an important factor in decreasing heavy bleeding by regulating excessive estrogen levels. Turmeric, or curcumin, is also used to promote liver health in traditional medicine. Research suggests that it has antibacterial properties. Turmeric is a delicious herb often used for flavoring in traditional Indian dishes. Silymarin, or milk thistle, protects liver functions through its flavonoid content. These herbs are all strong antioxidants and help protect the liver from damage.

CHAPTER 9

Menopause

Menopause officially begins after a woman's last menstrual period. However, most people use this word to describe the symptoms that a woman experiences during her late forties, fifties, and even sixties, as her female hormones decrease to a much lower level than she had during her active reproductive years. The loss of female hormones has a profound effect on the health of many tissues of the body. Here are the most common menopause symptoms and the vitamins, minerals, and herbs that are useful in preventing and relieving these symptoms.

Common Menopause Symptoms

The most frequently experienced symptoms of menopause are listed below.

Hot Flashes

Hot flashes and other vasomotor symptoms are women's most common complaints surrounding menopause. In fact, 80 percent of American women experience hot flashes, 40 percent of which are severe enough to require medical care. This high incidence of hot flashes is seen in menopausal women throughout the Western world, including Canada and Europe.

Many women can sense an oncoming hot flash seconds before it starts. Most describe the hot flash as a sudden and intense episode of warmth and heat. These episodes may take place unexpectedly, with a woman suddenly noticing that she feels warm and wants to remove a sweater or jacket. The hot flashes usually begin above the waist, especially on the chest, face, and neck, and then radiate to other parts of the body. The blood vessels of the skin dilate when the hot flash is occurring, causing the skin to become pink or rose-colored.

The hot flashes are often accompanied by varying amounts of sweating—mild in some women, profuse in others. Women with more severe episodes may become so wet that they have to change their clothes or bed sheets. After being first too warm, skin temperature then cools down from sweating and causes shivering. This temperature instability can be very uncomfortable for many women, forcing them to alternately shed and then add clothes. Studies have recorded measurable changes in skin temperature just before the hot flash begins. In addition, there is a 10 to 15 percent increase in pulse rate.

The hot flash usually lasts from 30 seconds to 5 minutes. However, in extreme cases, patients report hot flashes lasting as long as an hour. Frequency also varies. Some notice them infrequently, having only a few a year or once or twice a month. Many women will have hot flashes on a daily basis: three or four episodes a day are not unusual, and, in severe cases, 30 to

40 hot flashes occurring in a day. Other women may have several hot flashes during the night. This can disrupt their sleep and cause their spouse to wake up, too, because of the profuse perspiration and discomfort.

Women who have hot flashes often have other symptoms, as well. Like hot flashes, these symptoms are due to vasomotor instability and, thus, are believed to arise from the same cause. These symptoms may present odd sensations that can be quite worrisome to women who do not understand that they are menopause-related; but for most women, they diminish in time. They include nausea, dizziness, faintness, and palpitations (rapid and forceful heartbeats). Some women notice numbness and tingling in their arms and fingers. And some even experience formication, a crawling feeling over the skin.

When hot flashes occur throughout the night, they often disturb sleep. Many women wake up feeling hot and perspiring profusely. Often it is difficult to go back to sleep and women feel exhausted the next day. Sleep-deprivation insomnia is a common reason why menopausal women visit their doctors seeking relief.

Fortunately, symptoms of hot flashes do not last forever. For half of all menopausal women, the hot flash symptoms disappear within a year. For another 30 percent of women, they last up to two and a half years. Unfortunately, however, for 20 percent of women, the hot flashes and other vasomotor symptoms can last 5 to 10 years or even longer.

Vaginal and Bladder Aging

With the onset of menopause, estrogen levels can drop as much as 75 percent. Estrogen causes dilation and relaxation of the blood vessels, promoting good circulation to the body's organs and tissues. When the estrogen levels dwindle, blood flow to the genitals decreases. The tissues lose their pink or rosy color and, over time, become more pale. The vagina has many estrogen receptors, so the vaginal tissues are very responsive to the levels of hormones available. When estrogen is deficient, the vaginal and urethral linings lose their thick protective layer of surface cells and become thinner, drier, and less elastic. The cervix and vagina secrete less mucous. As a result, they are much more easily injured and traumatized.

Early signs of vaginal and bladder aging are, unfortunately, not the only ones. In time, the vagina actually shrinks and becomes much shorter and narrower at the opening. The vaginal walls become less elastic.

As you can imagine, these changes in the vagina and bladder cause uncomfortable symptoms and affect a woman's ability to function normally.

Vaginal Soreness and Painful Intercourse

As the vagina thins and narrows it can become easily irritated and sore from penetration in any form. Many women find that their annual pelvic examination and PAP smear become quite an ordeal. The introduction of a vaginal speculum can be painful. Sexual activity can be equally uncomfortable. The thrusting of the penis inside an atrophied vagina can cause excessive friction and discomfort. Many women experience a mild burning sensation with sexual activity.

Loss of Sexual Desire

The vaginal pain and discomfort due to atrophic changes can cause a loss of sexual desire. Until the problem is treated and solved, some women, not surprisingly, try to avoid sex. Even women who formerly enjoyed sex may make excuses or keep away from intimate situations where they might engage in sexual activity.

In addition to the actual physical changes that make sexual activity uncomfortable, lack of hormonal support also decreases sexual arousal and sexual desire. Many postmenopausal women report a decrease in frequency and intensity of orgasm. Clitoral sensitivity can diminish, as does the sensitivity of the cervix to deep thrusting of the penis. Many of these changes are due to decreased estrogen stimulation of the nerve cells and blood vessels. Both nerve cells and blood vessels contain high levels of estrogen receptors. Lack of estrogen causes poor circulation to the genital region and decreased nerve response during sexual intercourse (or any sexual activity).

Loss of testosterone also decreases sexual desire or libido. Testosterone is produced during our active reproductive years by both the ovaries and the adrenals. Ten to 20 percent of women experience a drop in libido rather soon after ceasing menstruation. This is because their ovaries stop making testosterone as well as estrogen. (In other women, the drop in testosterone may not occur until some years after menopause. As a result, their sexual desire may not decrease as rapidly.)

Vaginal and Bladder Infections

Vaginal infections can occur frequently in postmenopausal women because of the thinning and drying of the vaginal lining. The lining becomes easily irritated and injured. As a result, it becomes very susceptible to infections by unhealthy organisms such as yeast and bacteria. The lack of estrogen support also causes the vaginal pH to change from acidic to alkaline. When the pH becomes too alkaline, our normal healthy bacteria die off and are replaced by organisms that thrive in an alkaline pH. These organisms infect the tissues and cause unpleasant symptoms such as vaginal discharge, burning, and unpleasant odor.

Recurrent urinary tract infections can also be a difficult and unpleasant problem for postmenopausal women. In fact, the standard medical textbooks state that 10 percent of these women suffer from recurrent infections. Why do so many urinary tract infections occur? First, with the loss of estrogen support, the urethra, the small tube near the vaginal opening through which urine leaves the body, becomes less flexible and elastic. Like the vagina, its walls thin out and become drier. Because the urethra is located so near the vaginal opening, it can become easily irritated after sexual intercourse and thus, much more prone to infection. As women age, the lower urinary tract also stops manufacturing antiadherence factors, which help to prevent bacteria from attaching to the bladder wall. Common symptoms of urinary tract infection include frequency, burning, and itching upon urination. Women may have to urinate quite often, but void only a small amount of urine.

Menopausal Mood Swings

During the menopausal years women may notice that their moods fluctuate more easily. Mood changes can run the gamut from increased anxiety and irritability, to depression and fatigue. Many women become distressed by this tendency because it can affect the quality of their personal relationships. They report being much grouchier than usual towards family, friends, and co-workers and responding to daily life stresses more irritably.

Many women describe these feelings as being similar to the emotional ups-and-downs of Premenstrual Syndrome (PMS). In fact, a woman who has had bouts of PMS during her active reproductive years may be particularly distressed by her emotional fluctuations. Often, her expectation is that PMS symptoms will disappear, not be accentuated as she transitions into menopause.

For most women, the causes of the mood swings are complex and can be due to hormonal changes, social and cultural factors, or, more often, a combination of both. Some women are very sensitive to the rapid drop in estrogen and progesterone levels that occurs with menopause. They may feel like they are on an emotional rollercoaster as their hormones drop and readjust to a new, lower level. This is because estrogen and progesterone have a profound effect on the mood as well as the physical body. Progesterone acts as a sedative on the nervous system. When levels are too high, women may feel depressed and tired. Estrogen has more of a stimulatory effect on the nervous system, causing anxiety and irritability when estrogen output is elevated. (Conversely, women may feel more depressed and moody when estrogen levels are diminished).

Under optimal conditions, estrogen and progesterone output exists in a state of healthy equilibrium in the body. When we feel comfortable emotionally and are not experiencing extreme mood fluctuations, this equilibrium has probably been reached. However, with the transition into menopause, hormonal levels shift rapidly, fluctuating between very high and low levels, then occasionally settling into balance again. Finally, both hormones drop permanently to low, postmenopausal levels. The moods, likewise, may follow no obvious pattern in very sensitive women, fluctuating as hormones shift.

The social and cultural factors before, during, and after menopause may be quite stressful for some women and can contribute to mood fluctuations. For example, menopause can be a time when children leave home and move away, major career changes are made, and marriage ends in divorce or starts anew. The combination of hormonal and biochemical changes plus lifestyle changes can be quite difficult for many women to handle. Some women find themselves alone without their old, familiar support systems intact during this time of transition. Other women find that, in addition, they have to cope with their husbands' midlife crises, engendered by loss of job or job dissatisfaction, health problems, and other issues that commonly crop up for men at that time. At the very least, some women are emotionally distressed by the changes that menopause causes in their physical body. Many mention feeling unhappy with the wrinkles, loss of muscle tone, and change in body shape that can occur very rapidly after menopause.

Suggestions for Relief of Symptoms

What solutions are available for women who do need help in relieving their hot flashes, night sweats, vaginal and bladder symptoms, as well as mood instability during the early menopausal years?

1. **Hormone replacement therapy** (HRT), using a combination of estrogen and progesterone, can be a tremendous help for women with moderate to severe symptoms. HRT tends to act rapidly in many women to relieve symptoms, and is available in a variety of doses and delivery systems. Depending upon their symptoms women can choose readily from oral tablets, skin patches, and vaginal creams. Skin creams and gels are available, though infrequently prescribed, in the United States.

2. **Effective management of stress** can play an important role in relieving and preventing menopausal symptoms. Women with more frequent hot flashes and mood swings may find meditation, deep breathing exercises, yoga, and a variety of other relaxation techniques to be quite helpful in controlling their symptoms.

3. A change in diet can relieve symptoms. Certain foods also trigger hot flashes, dry out tissues, and can worsen mood. These include alcohol and caffeine-containing beverages like coffee, black tea, and cola drinks. Obviously, the intake of these foods should be avoided. Chocolate should be eliminated, too, since it contains caffeine. Its high-sugar content can also destabilize the blood sugar level. Some women need to avoid spicy foods if hot flashes are severe.

A low-fat, high-fiber diet with plenty of fresh fruits and vegetables, whole grains, legumes (beans and peas), raw seeds, and nuts is optimal. Meat intake, especially red meat, should be avoided or kept to a minimum since saturated fat is unhealthy for women as they age.

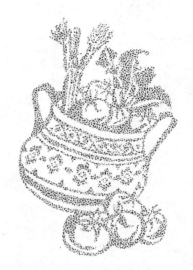

Vitamins and Minerals for Relief of Hot Flashes, Night Sweats, Vaginal and Bladder Atrophy

The following vitamins, minerals, and herbs can be helpful for relief of menopausal symptoms.

Vitamin A. Vitamin A is necessary for the growth and support of the skin, mucous membranes, and eyes. Deficiency of vitamin A causes night blindness; rough, scaly skin; fatigue; and increased susceptibility to infections. As a result, this nutrient is very important for the support of the vulvar, vaginal, and bladder tissues. In fact, lack of vitamin A is a risk factor for development of bladder and cervical cancer. A lack of adequate vitamin A can predispose a woman to skin conditions related to the aging process, such as vulvar leukoplakia and senile keratosis. Both of these conditions can precede the onset of cancer.

Vitamin A is best taken in the vegetable source, beta

carotene. This is because vitamin A from animal sources (usually fish liver oil) accumulates in the liver. If the vitamin A levels in the body become too high, headaches and liver toxicity can occur. Doses of more than 25,000 IU per day, if taken for periods longer than several months, are considered unsafe. However, the provitamin A beta carotene, which is derived from plant sources such as fruits and vegetables, is very safe for most women, even at higher doses. For women with vaginal and bladder atrophy, I generally recommend 25,000 to 100,000 IU per day. (25,000 IU of beta carotene is found in one sweet potato or one cup of carrot juice.) Thus, food can be a potent source of this nutrient.

Vitamin C. Vitamin C is found abundantly in nature. Many fruits and vegetables, as well as some meats, contain high levels of vitamin C. The body needs adequate amounts to maintain the skin, including the vulvar, vaginal, and bladder tissues. Vitamin C is necessary for collagen synthesis and skin strength. A low-vitamin C intake has been found to predispose women to cervical dysplasia and cancer of the cervix.

The diet of women with early-stage cervical cancer has been compared to those of healthy women in controlled research studies. The women with cervical cancer were found to have a diet much lower in foods containing vitamin C. While vitamin C alone will not reverse bladder and vaginal atrophy, sufficient daily intake of this nutrient is necessary along with vitamin A for the support of these tissues.

I generally recommend between 1000 to 5000 mg per day for menopausal women. Side effects are rare, although some women find that the higher doses cause diarrhea. If this happens to you, simply reduce the dose to a comfortable level. Rarely, large doses of vitamin C can predispose you to kidney stones. If you have a history of kidney stones, keep your vitamin C intake well below 5000 mg per day. If you have any questions about these issues, ask your physician. Millions of women do use vitamin C, even at high doses, with no side effects and derive many health benefits from its use.

Bioflavonoids. While bioflavonoids can help relieve and prevent premenopausal symptoms, they can be equally useful for menopausal women. This is because bioflavonoids are actually weakly estrogenic and can be used as a safe, nontoxic substitute for estrogen. Unlike the hormones prescribed for medical use, bioflavonoids contain low potencies (1/50,000 of that of stilbestrol, a synthetic estrogen), and have no side effects for most women. Bioflavonoids can help relieve hot flashes as well as vaginal dryness. One study of 94 women at Loyola University Medical School in 1964 showed a bioflavonoid-vitamin C combination to be effective in controlling hot flashes in most of the women tested. Interestingly, in this particular study, bioflavonoids were suggested as a possible estrogen substitute for cancer patients with estrogen-sensitive tumors who could not use hormone replacement therapy. In support of this recommendation, it is noteworthy that Japanese women have a low rate of breast cancer. Their customary soy-based diet (which is high in bioflavonoids) is actually thought to help protect them from developing this disease.

A diet containing soy and flax seed oil may also help protect women from developing vaginal atrophy. In one study reported in the *British Medical Journal* in 1990, supplementing the diet with soy flour and flax seed oil provided enough source of plant-based estrogen to actually help build up and thicken the vaginal lining. Women who don't want to eat a soy-based diet but want relief of the vaginal and hot flash symptoms can use bioflavonoids in a purified form as a nutritional supplement. The usual dose varies from 500 to 2000 mg.

Vitamin E. There is a long history of research studies that have found vitamin E to reduce menopausal symptoms. Some of the studies date back as far as forty and fifty years ago. This nutrient has shown promise as a useful treatment for hot flashes, night sweats, and even vaginal dryness. Depending on the study, between 66 to 85 percent of the women tested found vitamin E to be an effective substitute for estrogen. Vitamin E can be a good treatment option for women who cannot or do not want to use the higher potencies of prescription hormones. For example, one 1945 study in the *American Journal of Obstetrics and Gynecology* reported that nearly all of 25 cancer patients showed an excellent response to the use of vitamin E therapy. These women had become menopausal either through surgical or radiation therapy for their cancers. All the women studied had severe hot flashes and mood alterations that could not be treated by estrogen replacement therapy due to their types of tumors. Using vitamin E as an estrogen substitute, 23 out of the 25 women had either complete relief or significant improvement of their symptoms.

Another interesting study of 47 menopausal women published in the *British Medical Journal* in 1943 found that vitamin E not only helped reduce hot flashes in 64 percent of the women tested but also helped reduce symptoms of vaginal aging. Fifty percent of the women noted healing of vaginal atrophy as well as a decrease in pain on sexual intercourse. Many women with vaginal atrophy are also prone to recurrent vaginal infections which produce uncomfortable symptoms like itching, burning, and discharge. A 1954 study in the *American Journal of Obstetrics and Gynecology* reported that 44 women at high risk of developing yeast vaginitis because of a preexisting diabetic condition noted significant relief of symptoms when treated with vitamin E vaginal suppositories.

Generally, I recommend that women take between 400 to

2400 IU of vitamin E per day beginning at a low-dose level and increasing the dosage gradually over several weeks until the desired symptom relief is achieved. Women with hypertension, diabetes, or bleeding problems, however, should begin at much lower dosages of vitamin E (100 IU per day). If you have any of these conditions, ask your physician about the advisability of using vitamin E. In general, however, vitamin E tends to be well tolerated and is used by millions of people without adverse effects. Many patients with severe vaginal atrophy use vitamin E topically. Besides taking vitamin E orally, women can open a capsule and apply the oil directly to the vaginal tissues. Vitamin E occurs abundantly in vegetable oils, raw nuts, and seeds, and in some fruits and vegetables.

Essential Fatty Acids. These oils are particularly important to menopausal women because the deficiency of these oils is responsible, in part, for the drying of tissues at midlife: the vaginal and bladder mucosa, as well as the skin, and hair. The lack of sufficient fatty acids at menopause is a nutritional problem because they cannot be made by the body and must be supplied daily in the diet. The main sources of essential fatty acids are raw seeds and nuts or fish. Unfortunately, these foods are not a staple of the typical American (or Western) diet.

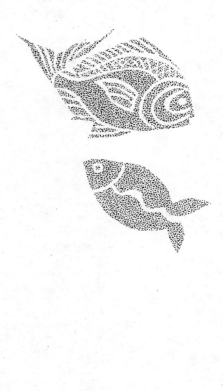

Along with vitamin E and bioflavonoids, which can also promote a build-up of the vaginal lining, I recommend these oils extensively in my nutritional programs for women. Both the whole ground flax seeds (which are 50 percent oil) and the purified oil in capsule form are excellent sources of the two essential oils, linoleic acid and linolenic acid. Though flax seed oil was used as a food supplement in the study of vaginal atrophy reported in the *British Medical Journal* in 1990, many women prefer to take the essential fatty acids in capsule form. Other excellent sources of essential fatty acids include evening primrose oil, borage oil, and black currant oil. Unlike flax oil, none of these other oils are actually used as food. They are used primarily as nutritional supplements. I find that 2 to 8 capsules per day is a helpful dose, at least in the early stages when trying to replace moisture and softness in the skin. Alternatively, women who like the buttery taste of raw flax oil may want to take 1 to 3 tablespoons per day.

Herbs for Reduction of Menopausal Hot Flashes, Night Sweats, Vaginal and Bladder Atrophy

Phytoestrogens. Phytoestrogen plants abound in nature. They contain estrogen similar to the hormones manufactured by our own body. Many of these plants can actually be used as an estrogen substitute by women who cannot or do not want to use estrogen in pharmacological (or drug) dosages. This can be the case with women who have preexisting health problems, such as migraine headaches or hypertension, or who are sensitive to the dosages used in standard hormone replacement therapy. Phytoestrogen herbs provide a helpful alternative for these women.

Compared with drug potencies, plant sources of estrogen are very weak. Other estrogen-containing plants besides bioflavonoids, like fennel and anise, licorice-flavored kitchen herbs, have been assayed as 1/400 the potency of estradiol, the main form of estrogen made by the ovaries. Because of their weak potencies, estrogen-containing herbs tend to have a low potential for causing side effects, yet are quite effective in suppressing such common menopausal symptoms as hot flashes and night sweats. They can even help build up the vaginal walls, which tend to thin and atrophy due to estrogen deficiency. Other plant sources of estrogen and progesterone used in traditional herbology include dong quai, black cohosh, blue cohosh, unicorn root, false unicorn root, sarsaparilla.

Wild yam, which comes from barbasco root (a giant, wild yam grown in Mexico) has been found to contain natural plant sources of DHEA (dehydroepiandrosterone). DHEA is the precursor to all our male and female hormones. Many women are now using wild yams as a natural source of plant hormones to help control hot flashes and other postmenopausal symptoms.

Plants may also form the basis for the production of medical hormones. Many common plants such as soybeans and yams contain a preformed steroidal nucleus. Estrogen and progesterone can be synthesized from plants in relatively few steps and have enabled sex hormones to become available commercially at a reasonable cost.

Antibiotic Herbs. Women who suffer from vaginal and bladder atrophy due to estrogen deficiency run the additional risk of increased incidence of infections in these tissues. The tissues become more delicate and easily traumatized after menopause. Many herbs appear to have an ability to soothe, relieve irritation, and reduce infection in the urinary tract, including goldenseal, uva ursi, blackberry root, and wintergreen. Goldenseal contains berberine, an alkaloid with antibiotic activity. It may also help to combat vaginitis due to yeast infections, a great problem for many postmenopausal women. Uva ursi contains allantoin (a chemical that helps to promote new cell growth), chemical diuretics, and antioinfective agents.

CHAPTER 10

Osteoporosis, Heart Disease, and Breast Cancer

The decrease in hormones that occurs soon after menopause can cause a number of uncomfortable symptoms, but the long-term effects of hormonal loss can produce devastating (and potentially life-threatening) consequences. Estrogen protects the heart and bones from aging. With the loss of this hormone, the incidence of osteoporosis and heart attacks increases with age in high-risk women. Breast cancer also occurs much more commonly in postmenopausal women, since immune function diminishes with age. This chapter presents basic facts about these three postmenopausal health problems and offers suggestions for vitamins, minerals, and herbs which can help to prevent them.

Osteoporosis

One of the most serious consequences of postmenopausal aging is the development of osteoporosis. In fact, osteoporosis is a major health problem affecting more than 20 million older Americans, 90 percent of whom are women. One out of three American women will develop osteoporosis after menopause.

The statistics surrounding osteoporosis are astounding. More than 1.3 million fractures occur in the United States each year because of this condition, including 250,000 hip fractures. Eighty percent of these fractures occur in women over 65 with osteoporosis. About one-quarter of these women die within one year from complications caused by their fractures, such as blood clots and pneumonia. Another one-third never regain the ability to function physically or socially on their own. These women spend the rest of their lives requiring long-term care in nursing facilities. Besides causing hip fractures, osteoporosis is also responsible for loss of bone in the jaw, gum recession (both of which are early signs of this condition), dowager's humps, loss of height, back pain due to compression and fractures of the vertebra, and fractures of the wrist (known as *colles fractures* by physicians).

Often these fractures occur in situations that put only mild stress on the bone, and would not normally cause such an outcome. This can include missing a step and falling down, falling on an extended arm, or lifting a heavy object. Because of the underlying weakness of the bone, fractures can also occur spontaneously without any preceding trauma. This is often the case with vertebral fractures.

Risk Factors for Osteoporosis

Not all women have the same risk of developing osteoporosis. Some women maintain strong and heavy bones throughout their lives, while other women develop accelerated bone loss soon after menopause. If you suspect you are at higher risk of developing osteoporosis, become knowledgeable about which factors have actually been linked to a higher incidence of this disease. This will help you and your physician evaluate your own risk when planning an optimal treatment program. These factors include racial background, family history, hormonal status, lifestyle habits, and preexisting health conditions.

RACIAL BACKGROUND

Skin pigmentation appears to correlate with bone mass. Black women are less likely to develop osteoporosis than white women. In fact, women at the highest risk are small and fair-skinned. These are typically women of northern European ancestry such as Dutch, German, or English background with blond, reddish, or light brown hair and pale skin. Asian women also have a higher risk of developing osteoporosis.

FAMILY HISTORY

If your close female relatives suffered from osteoporosis, you run a higher risk of developing this problem. Many women have seen their own mothers or grandmothers develop a dowager's hump or become disabled from fracturing their hips. This can be quite upsetting for the entire family who must deal with the long-term disability.

HORMONAL STATUS

The age at which women begin menopause and how much hormonal support they maintain during their postmenopausal years affects bone density. Women who have had a surgical menopause before the age of 40, with removal of their ovaries, are at high risk of developing osteoporosis because of the abrupt withdrawal of estrogen at a young age. Similarly, women who go through an early natural menopause are at high risk of osteoporosis. A woman going through early menopause at age 35 or 40 has as much as 10 to 15 years less estrogen protection of her bones than a woman going through menopause at age 50. Thus, the older you are when going through menopause, the more years of hormonal protection you provide for your bones.

While obesity is a health risk for many diseases such as osteoarthritis and uterine cancer, being overweight does confer some protection against osteoporosis in postmenopausal women. This is because the fat cells produce estrone, a type of estrogen, through conversion of the adrenal hormone androstenedione. This type of estrogen does provide some support for the bones once the ovarian source of estrogen has dwindled.

LIFESTYLE HABITS

Women who engage in regular physical exercise and are more muscular have a lower risk of developing osteoporosis. Physical activity helps keep women flexible and agile, which also reduces the likelihood of fractures. Conversely, inactivity increases the risk. Even young men or women confined to bed for long periods of time show a decrease in bone mass.

Many nutritional factors affect the risk of developing osteoporosis. Women who drink more than two cups of coffee per day or excessive amounts of other caffeine containing beverages like black tea or colas, or consume more than two alcoholic drinks per day are at higher risk. High-protein or high-salt intake are risk factors, as is inadequate calcium intake. Smokers also run a higher risk of osteoporosis.

Women with a history of bulimia, anorexia, or malabsorption syndrome run a higher risk of poor calcium absorption or low-estrogen levels. This is often the case in women with anorexia who don't have enough body fat to produce adequate estrogen. Women who use thyroid medication, or cortisone for a variety of conditions or who suffer from an overactive thyroid gland are at higher risk. This is also true of women with chronic kidney disease. All of these conditions can adversely affect the calcium balance in the body.

DIAGNOSIS OF OSTEOPOROSIS

Excellent tests now exist to evaluate the likelihood of developing osteoporosis. They also allow physicians to diagnose osteoporosis in the early stages before the bone loss is so severe that it causes fractures. These tests include the single-photon densitometer, which measures the density of the forearm bone; the dual photon densitometer, which measures the spine or hip bone; and the computerized axial topography scan (also called a CAT scan), which measures bone density in the spine. The CAT scan uses higher amounts of X rays and is a more expensive test. These tests are much more sensitive than the conventional X ray, which picks up osteoporosis only when 30 percent or more of the bone mass is lost.

You may want to have a bone density test if you are trying to decide whether or not to use hormonal replacement therapy (HRT). If the tests show accelerated bone loss for your age group, you should seriously consider the use of HRT unless other major health issues contraindicate the use of hormones. The use of estrogen and progesterone, in combination, not only help to retain calcium in the bones, but appear to promote the growth of new bone. A vegetarian-based diet is optimal for prevention of osteoporosis. A diet high in meat tends to promote loss of calcium from the body.

Heart Disease

Cardiovascular disease is the major cause of death for American women, claiming the lives of half a million women per year. This is twice the number of women who die from cancer per year. While younger women do die of heart disease, it is a rare occurrence; the numbers tend to escalate as women age. Cancer is the main cause of death in women from age 30 to 60 (with heart disease in second place from age 40 to 60). Heart disease becomes the leading cause of death in women by age 60.

Most women die from heart attacks due to coronary artery disease. With coronary artery disease, there is a narrowing of one or more of the arteries that supply blood and oxygen to the heart. This narrowing is due to the formation of plaque in the arteries. Plaque is a thick, waxy, yellowish substance consisting primarily of cholesterol, smooth muscle cells, and foam cells. As the formation of plaque progresses, it can obstruct the flow of blood through the blood vessels. Over time, this can seriously compromise the function of the heart, finally leading to a heart attack. Unfortunately, the obstruction is usually quite advanced before it even begins to cause symptoms. Usually the symptoms consist of chest pain (angina) and shortness of breath on mild exertion.

Risk Factors for Heart Disease

Much research has been done over the past few decades to determine if certain women run a higher risk of developing heart disease. A number of studies have pinpointed factors that appear to be linked to a higher likelihood of developing this disease. These include specific physical characteristics: health factors such as family history, blood lipid profile, hypertension, and diabetes; and lifestyle factors such as smoking, lack of activity, and stress.

PHYSICAL CHARACTERISTICS

Age. As mentioned earlier, the older the woman, the greater her risk of developing heart disease. The highest incidence is in women over 65 years of age.

Body Weight. Women who are between 20 to 30 percent over their ideal weight are considered to be at greater risk of developing heart disease. This was noted in a study done by Harvard Medical School, which tested more than 115,000 women over eight years. Excess weight was found to be a significant factor in women developing coronary artery disease during the period of the study.

Body Shape—Distribution of Fat. Not only is overall obesity a risk factor, but how fat is distributed on the body affects heart disease risk, too. Women who distribute their excess weight in their middle or are rounder, shaped like apples, have a higher risk of coronary artery disease than pear-shaped women who distribute their fat in their hips and thighs.

HEALTH FACTORS

Family History of Heart Disease. You are at higher risk of developing heart disease if your close relatives have had a heart attack at an early age. Statistically, your risk is increased if your father had a heart attack before age 56 or your mother before age 60. Similarly, you are at a higher risk if your grandparents had a heart attack at a young age.

Blood Lipid Profile. Triglycerides are the form in which fat is stored in the body's tissues: three fatty acid molecules hooked to a glycerol backbone. Women with *Elevated triglyc-erides*, or triglycerides elevated in the blood to a level of 190 md/dl or greater, run a higher risk of developing coronary artery disease.

Elevated total cholesterol and LDL cholesterol. Cholesterol is a yellowish, waxy substance manufactured in our body primar-ily by the liver and, to a lesser extent, by the intestines. We also ingest cholesterol when we eat dairy products or red meat. How effectively cholesterol is used depends upon how effi-ciently it is transported throughout the body and how well the body can store or dispose of any excess. Transportation in the body is potentially a problem because the fatty cholesterol isn't soluble in blood, which is mostly water. To solve this problem, the body packages the cholesterol with a protein that allows the fat to be mixed with the blood. This process takes place in the liver, where several types of cholesterol-protein mixtures are produced.

The major type of cholesterol-protein manufactured is the low-density lipoprotein, or LDL. LDL is the body's main car-rier of cholesterol. When levels of LDL are elevated they re-main in the body streams and injure the endothelium (the inner lining of the blood vessel wall), thereby initiating plaque formation. Thus, LDL is considered to be the "bad" type of cholesterol. Women with a total blood cholesterol above 240 mg/dl and a LDL level above 160 mg/dl are thought to be at high risk of heart disease. Ideally, the total cholesterol should be below 180 mg/dl and the LDL below 130 mg/dl for the greatest degree of protection.

Decreased HDL cholesterol. The liver also makes another type of cholesterol-protein called the high-density lipoprotein or HDL. The HDL is considered to be the "good" type of choles-terol. This is because HDL picks up and carries the excess cho-lesterol back to the liver, where it is secreted into the bile. The bile empties the excess cholesterol into the intestinal tract, where it is excreted from our bodies through bowel movements. When her HDL is less than 35 mg/dl, a woman is considered to be at high risk of coronary artery disease. The HDL should ideally be about 55 mg/dl.

Elevated LDL to HDL ratio. The ratio between the LDL and HDL is also an important indicator of heart disease risk. Ideally, your LDL to HDL ratio should be no higher than 4:1. For example, if your HDL is 30 and your LDL is 150, then your ratio is 5:1, which puts you in the high-risk category.

Hypertension. High blood pressure is a significant risk factor for developing coronary artery disease. Sixty million Americans have elevated blood pressure readings, and nearly half of these people are women. Blood pressure is considered to be elevated when readings are above 140/90. The upper number is called the systolic pressure, which is the pressure that occurs when the heart contracts and pushes blood through the arterial circulation. The bottom number is called the diastolic blood pressure. This is the pressure in the arteries when the heart relaxes between beats. Not only does hypertension increase the likelihood of heart attacks, but it also increases the risk of strokes and kidney disease.

Diabetes. The Framingham Study, an important study of cardiovascular disease risk that has been ongoing in Massachusetts since 1949, found that women with diabetes are twice as likely to have a heart attack as nondiabetic women. Diabetic women are also at higher risk of developing serious visual problems and kidney complications, as well as hypertension and higher cholesterol levels.

LIFESTYLE FACTORS

Cigarette Smoking. Because smoking narrows the diameter of the blood vessels, impairing circulation, smokers have an increased risk of heart attacks and strokes. Smokers are also more likely to have higher levels of the bad LDL and lower levels of the good HDL. Unfortunately, 27 percent of all women smoke and this percentage is not declining rapidly, despite the great amount of public information on the health perils of smoking. Women smokers also enter menopause two to three years earlier than nonsmokers.

Physical Inactivity. Women with sedentary lifestyles have three times the risk of developing heart disease than women who are physically active. The heart is a muscle that needs to be exercised. Women who engage in aerobic exercise, such as walking at least three times a week for a half hour, have lower resting heart rate, greater lung capacity, and an improved ability to handle stress.

Stress. Several studies suggest that severe stress is a risk factor in developing coronary artery disease, though this link has been researched much less in women than in men. Many studies have been done on the Type A, hard-driving, aggressive male personality. However, women with multiple home and work responsibilities are often as hard-driving and stressed as men. This can predispose certain women over time to an increased risk of heart attack.

FEMALE-RELATED RISK FACTORS

Menopausal Status. The risk of coronary artery disease increases twofold to threefold once a woman enters natural menopause. Research studies, including the Framingham Study, have confirmed that premenopausal women with intact ovarian function enjoy significant protection against the development of heart attacks.

Surgical or Natural Menopause Before Age 45. Recent studies have shown that women who, during their premenopausal years, undergo a hysterectomy involving removal of their ovaries have three times the risk of coronary artery disease compared to women who cease menstruating at a later age. Similarly, a study of 122,000 nurses found that women who went through surgical menopause before the age of 35 have two to seven times the risk of heart attack. The risk is also higher in women who go through natural menopause at an early age. Estrogen appears to confer significant protection against heart attacks during the active reproductive years. The longer a woman menstruates, the more years her vascular system has estrogenic protection.

Hormonal Therapy for Heart Disease Prevention. Both estrogen alone and combined estrogen-progestin therapy have been studied for the effects on the cardiovascular system. Estrogen appears to be beneficial; it lowers the levels of LDL cholesterol, which is linked to heart attacks, and raises the level of HDL cholesterol, which appears to confer protection. The one negative factor noted on studies of estrogen users was a moderate rise in triglycerides. On the other hand, however, physicians believe the use of estrogen will confer protection against heart attacks. The addition of progesterone to an estrogen treatment program does not appear to negate estrogen's positive effects on the heart.

Breast Cancer

The incidence of breast cancer has increased dramatically over the past two decades. During the 1950s, it was estimated that one out of every twenty Americans would develop this disease. These estimates have been revised many times over the past forty years as the incidence of breast cancer has skyrocketed. It is currently estimated that one out of eight women, or

12 percent of all women in this country, will develop breast cancer during her lifetime. This is a staggering number, placing breast cancer as the most common cancer of American women today. It is the second most common cause of cancer deaths in women, behind only lung cancer in its mortality rate. In absolute numbers, 180,000 new cases of breast cancer were projected for 1993, as well as 46,000 deaths from this disease.

Breast cancer cells, like other malignancies, invade and destroy normal tissue (unlike benign tumors, which remain confined within a specific area). Breast cancer cells first grow within the breast tissue itself. In the later stages of the disease, the cancerous cells spread to other parts of the body near or adjacent to the breast (as with invasion to the lymph nodes). The cancerous cells can also invade distant sites, like the liver and the bones.

How high a woman's chance of survival is depends on how early the cancer is detected. The earlier the detection and the more localized a tumor is to the breast tissue itself, the more likely a woman is to have a long-term recovery from this disease (five years or more). For example, women with localized tumors are eight times more likely to survive the disease long-term than a woman with an advanced case that has spread throughout her body.

Risk Factors for Breast Cancer

Not all women have the same risk of developing breast cancer. While any woman can develop the disease, certain factors do put some women statistically at greater risk:

- Previous history of breast cancer.
- Family history of breast cancer. This is particularly pertinent if a woman's mother or sisters had the disease.

- Early onset of menstrual periods.
- Late menopause. Women who menstruate for more than 40 years seem to be at particular risk of breast cancer.
- Postmenopausal age—most breast cancers occur after age 50.
- Childlessness or having a first child after age 30.
- Bottle feeding—women who nurse their children appear to be at lower risk.
- Certain types of "atypical" cell patterns with benign (noncancerous) breast disease.
- High-fat diet—this seems to be a risk factor for some cases of breast cancer.
- Obesity—a high-fat and too-rich diet causes women to be overweight, which is a risk factor for the development of this disease.
- Alcohol use—more than nine drinks per week significantly increases the risk.
- Height or tallness is a risk factor.
- Affluence or degree of wealth.
- Radiation exposure.
- Prolonged estrogen and progesterone use (this is still a controversial area in medicine, with some studies supporting this view and other studies contradicting it).
- Urban lifestyle.

Diagnosis of Breast Cancer

Breast cancer is often discovered by the woman herself on breast examination or by her physician during a medical visit. A woman can usually feel a hard, nontender mass that is not particularly movable within her breast tissue. Other signs of breast cancer can include swelling, dimpling, or redness of the breast tissue. If the cancer has spread to the lymph nodes under the armpit or above the collarbone, they may feel enlarged and hard.

Mammography, or an X ray of the breast, is a tremendously helpful diagnostic tool to pinpoint breast cancer. In fact, many early-stage cancers, too small to be felt manually, can be detected by mammography. As a matter of fact, it can detect 90 percent of all breast cancers. Undoubtedly, the use of mammography has saved many women's lives through early detection. Other techniques such as thermography, which detects heat changes in the breast tissue, and ultrasound, which uses high-frequency sound waves, are diagnostic tools used less often.

Despite the usefulness of all of these techniques, the definitive diagnosis of breast cancer can only be made by doing a surgical biopsy. This allows the tissue sample removed from the breast to be looked at under the microscope and examined for cancerous cells.

Once breast cancer is diagnosed, many treatment options are available. These include surgery and removal of the breast and lymph nodes, if indicated. Less radical surgery, which leaves the breast intact, is being used more for localized cancer. Radiation therapy and chemotherapy are also used with various treatment regimens. What regimen is finally selected depends on how localized or disseminated the tumor is, as well as the preference of the patient and physician. Women interested in prevention should follow a diet low in saturated fat and limit their alcohol intake.

Vitamins and Minerals for Prevention of Osteoporosis

These are nutrients that can be of help in promoting prevention:

Calcium. There are dozens of studies that reinforce the importance of calcium for the prevention of osteoporosis. Calcium is the most abundant mineral in the body, and 99 percent of it is deposited in the bones and teeth. (The other 1 percent of calcium is involved in blood clotting, nerve and muscle stimulation, and other important functions.) As a result, calcium is the most important structural mineral in bone. Along with phosphorus, calcium helps to build and maintain strong and healthy bones. However, calcium absorption becomes much less efficient by the time women reach their postmenopausal years due to the aging of the digestive tract. Calcium needs an acid environment in the stomach for proper digestion. As many as 40 percent of postmenopausal women lack sufficient stomach acid for proper calcium absorption.

Unfortunately, most women have too little calcium intake in their diets. The average American woman takes in 400 to 500 mg per day. This is far less than the recommended daily allowance (RDA) of 800 mg per day for women during their active reproductive years and the 1200 to 1500 mg per day needed by postmenopausal women.

As a result, adequate calcium supplementation is of major importance to prevent bone loss. The type of calcium used must be considered, also. The main type of calcium used in supplements has been calcium carbonate. This is an alkaline form of calcium and isn't absorbed well by some women. In contrast, calcium citrate, an acidified form of calcium, is well absorbed and a good source of this nutrient for women. Be sure to check the label of any calcium supplement to make sure the dosages and the type of calcium used are optimal for your needs.

Phosphorus. Phosphorus is the second most abundant mineral in the body, found in bones and soft tissues. A major structural mineral of bone, it is present in a specific ratio of 2.5 parts calcium to 1 part phosphorus. This balance is important for both minerals to be used efficiently by the body. Because the American diet contains abundant phosphorous in foods such as meat, eggs, grains, seeds, nuts, and soft drinks, phosphorus deficiency is relatively rare. In addition, phosphorus is easily absorbed from the digestive tract, with an absorption rate of approximately 70 percent. The RDA for phosphorus is 800 mg.

Magnesium. This is another important mineral for healthy bones. While not as prevalent as either calcium or phosphorus in bone, it is equally important. Magnesium is needed for bone growth, as well as for proper calcium absorption and assimilation. If the body has too little magnesium available, it deposits calcium pathologically in tissues and organs, so calcium accumulates in the muscles, heart, and kidneys. In susceptible women, calcium deposited in the kidneys can cause kidney stones. Therefore, a woman who increases her calcium intake should also increase magnesium intake in a ratio of 2:1 or 10:4 calcium to magnesium. Other minerals, like zinc, copper, manganese, and silicon, are also needed in trace amounts for healthy bone growth and regulation of bone metabolism.

Vitamin D. This fat-soluble vitamin can either be ingested in the diet or formed on the skin by exposure to sunlight. Sunlight activates a type of cholesterol found in the skin, converting it to vitamin D. Vitamin D is usually included in multivitamin products and is also found in fish liver oil supplements, along with vitamin A and fortified milk.

Vitamin D helps prevent osteoporosis by aiding in the absorption of calcium from the intestinal tract. It is needed for the synthesis of enzymes found in mucous membranes, which are, in turn, needed for the active transport of calcium. It also helps break down and assimilate phosphorus. A deficiency of vitamin D causes inadequate absorption of calcium from the intestinal tract and retention of phosphorus by the kidneys. This causes an imbalance in the calcium-phosphorus ratio, leading to faulty mineralization of the bones. Menopausal women should be sure to take the RDA of 400 IU per day of vitamin D.

Herbs for Prevention of Osteoporosis

Herbs as Mineral Sources. While they are not the primary source of calcium and other minerals for most women, herbs can still provide a valuable source of minerals along with other foods in the diet. Certain plants like kelp and other sea vegetables, as well as dandelion root, horsetail, and oat straw, are good sources of calcium, magnesium, and trace minerals needed for strong and healthy bones. Kelp and the other sea vegetables can be used as condiments to flavor food such as soups, casseroles, and salads. The other herbs may be taken in capsule form as supplements.

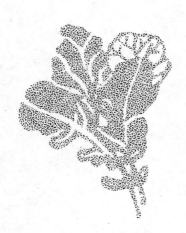

Vitamins and Minerals for Cardiovascular Disease Prevention

Beta Carotene. Oxygen-related damage to LDL cholesterol has been linked to the development of cardiovascular disease. Laboratory testing and a few clinical studies suggest that beta carotene can prevent this oxygen-related damage and, thereby, help protect the blood vessels from the disease process. It does this by inactivating singlet oxygen, a form of oxygen that is unstable and attacks cells in the body to gain a second electron. While the protective benefits of beta carotene have not been definitively proven, the studies to date suggest that its use may be beneficial in preventing heart disease. The U.S. Physicians' Health Study found that in a group of 333 participants with chest pain but no prior history of heart attack, beta carotene appeared to have a protective effect (with 50 percent fewer major cardiovascular events, such as heart attacks, strokes, and cardiac related deaths). I recommend the use of beta carotene or beta carotene-containing foods because of its many benefits for good health, aside from any possible cardiovascular protection.

Vitamin C. Like beta carotene, vitamin C is a water-soluble vitamin that appears to be helpful in preventing LDL cholesterol oxidation, a process which can initiate atherogenesis (the destruction of the blood vessel wall and the formation of plaque) and eventually, major incidents like heart attacks and strokes. In the recent Nurses' Health Study, sponsored by Harvard University, in which over 87,000 women between the ages of 34 and 54 were tested, the association between dietary intake of vitamin C and the risk of developing coronary artery disease was evaluated. The risk of developing heart disease was at least 42 percent lower for women who took high doses of vitamin C than for women with a low vitamin C intake. Another study done in the Boston area found that both male and female users of vitamin C supplementation had lower levels of blood pressure, lower LDL cholesterol, and higher levels of HDL cholesterol (the type of cholesterol that confers protection against coronary artery disease) than participants with a lower vitamin C intake. Vitamin C is also necessary for the regeneration of vitamin E in the body, another important antioxidant nutrient. These results make a good case for vitamin C's cardiovascular protective effects.

Vitamin E. This nutrient completes the triumvirate of antioxidant vitamins that appear to confer protection against cardiovascular disease. Vitamin E is the main fat-soluble antioxidant nutrient in the body. It lodges within the membranes inside and surrounding the cells, protecting the body against attack by singlet (unstable) oxygen and other free radicals that cause cell destruction. As mentioned earlier, singlet oxygen or other free radical destruction of LDL cholesterol may be one of the early steps leading to atherogenesis and ultimately, cardiovascular disease. Vitamin E, along with beta carotene and vitamin C, provides protection for both the water compartment as well as the fat compartment of our cells. This is necessary for the most complete protection against oxidative damage. Vitamin E also has a beneficial anticlotting effect on the blood. While a diet high in saturated fat diet tends to make blood cells become sticky and clump together, vitamin E causes the cells to disperse. This helps prevent blood clots from forming, an advantage for women past midlife who are at higher risk of stroke and heart attack.

Niacin. Niacin is a member of the vitamin B family which can cause blood vessels to dilate, producing a "niacin flush" whereby the user experiences a sensation of warmth, itching, and redness of the skin. As a vasodilator, niacin improves circulation to the arms and legs and helps to reduce blood pressure. It also lowers total blood cholesterol, a significant risk factor for heart attacks. Niacin also helps to improve the lipid profile by lowering bad LDL lipids and increasing the beneficial HDL cholesterol. To begin using niacin, start at 50 to 150 mg twice daily and increase slowly to 1500 to 2500 mg over a two to three month period. Be sure to use a B complex supplement containing the whole family of B vitamins when using niacin. (It is important to note that some women are never able to achieve high doses due to the severity of their niacin flush symptoms.)

Essential Fatty Acids. The supplemental use of Omega-3 fatty acids derived from fish oils like mackerel, salmon, and halibut, as well as plants like flax seed, pumpkin seed, and soybeans, have protective effects against cardiovascular disease. A number of studies have shown that these fatty acids can relax and dilate the blood vessels, as well as inhibit platelet cell aggregation (important in preventing clot formation). In addition, the Omega-3 fatty acids lower triglyceride level. This is beneficial because the elevation of triglycerides is a risk factor for coronary artery disease. However, the evidence for reduction of LDL cholesterol is not as conclusive. Also, since fish oil consumption can impair insulin secretion and increase blood glucose, its intake should be monitored in diabetics. Otherwise, the use of Omega-3 fatty acids may be a good idea for women wanting to prevent cardiovascular disease.

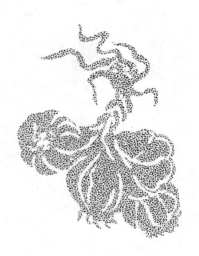

Herbs for Cardiovascular Disease Prevention

Anticlotting Herbs. Garlic and ginger are two delicious herbs which are used commonly as flavoring agents. They are also tremendously beneficial in reducing the risk of heart disease. Use the two plants if you have a strong family history of heart disease with early mortality (parents or siblings dying in their 50s or 60s of heart disease). They should also be used if you have many risk factors yourself, such as hypertension or elevated cholesterol. Both garlic and ginger have been researched for their ability to prevent aggregation or clotting of the blood. This is important for the prevention of strokes and heart attacks. In addition, both herbs help reduce cholesterol levels. Garlic has the additional benefit of reducing blood pressure.

If you find these foods too spicy for your taste, they can be taken in capsule form or as a liquid tincture. Women taking these herbs for cardiovascular disease prevention may want to eat several raw cloves of garlic a day or as many as 6 capsules of the herb used as a supplement. Take 4 capsules of ginger per day, if you do not use it as a food flavoring. However, you may find that 1 to 2 capsules per day suit your needs better.

Soluble Fibers. Fiber is the undigestible roughage found in many fruits, vegetables, and grains. Some fibers are important for their ability to bind fat and promote its excretion from the intestinal tract. Soluble fibers include oat bran, rice bran, pectin (found in apples), and guar gum which also helps to reduce sugar absorption from the intestines.

Vitamins and Minerals for Breast Cancer Prevention

Vitamin A. Beta carotene, the provitamin A found in fruits and vegetables, has been cited in a number of studies as an important nutrient in breast cancer prevention. In the Nurses' Health Study mentioned earlier, beta carotene proved protective against breast cancer for more than 87,000 women. A study published in 1992 by the State University of New York compared 310 women having breast cancer to 316 women without the disease. The study found that the cancer-free group ate many more beta carotene-containing fruits and vegetables than the women with breast cancer. In addition, the National Cancer Institute studied 83 women with breast cancer and found that they had lower blood levels of beta carotene. Beta carotene both in supplemental form and in foods like fresh fruits and vegetables should be included in your diet if you are interested in breast cancer prevention.

Vitamin C. In a 1991 review of 46 studies of the protective effect of vitamin C on cancer, in 33 studies vitamin C helped safeguard against the development of many cancers. This included nonhormone-dependent breast cancer. Vitamin C did not appear to confer any protection against hormone-dependent (including estrogen-dependent) breast cancers.

Fruits and vegetables are rich sources of both beta carotene and vitamin C. Supplemental vitamin C is helpful for women who want to lower their cancer risk for all types of cancer (including certain breast cancers).

Herbs for Breast Cancer Prevention

Anticancer Herbs. Many herbs show promise in the prevention and treatment of many human cancers, although their specific role in treating breast cancer is not clear. Herbs with possible anticancer activity include garlic, burdock root, alfalfa, and a host of others. One herb, in particular, may hold some promise for breast cancer prevention. This is red clover, an herb traditionally used by several different cultures to treat cancer. Research done at the National Cancer Institute has found anticarcinogenic compounds in red clover, including several bioflavonoids, genistein and daidzein, which are both weakly estrogenic and antiestrogenic (as described earlier in this book). Women who have preexisting breast cancer may want to check with their own physicians to see if red clover can be used safely as a nutritional adjunct to their regular medical program.

Two compounds that have been linked to a lower risk of breast cancer are bioflavonoids and lignans. Both are natural plant sources of very weak estrogens. Rich sources of bioflavonoids include soy, buckwheat, alfalfa sprouts, the inner peel of citrus fruits, and many berries. Lignans are particularly abundant in raw ground flax seed and are also found in whole grains and legumes. Diets that are rich in these foods seem to be a factor in preventing the development of breast cancer in women. There is also evidence to suggest that such a diet may help decrease the mortality rate of men from prostate cancer. In Asia, most notably in Japan, the rates of hormone-dependent cancers are significantly lower than those in Western Countries.

CHAPTER 11

Suggested Formulas and Vitamin Content of Foods

*I*n the previous chapters, I have included detailed information about nutrients for specific female health issues. Many women, however, have asked for information on how to combine these nutrients into multivitamin, mineral, and herbal formulas that they can use on a daily basis.

To respond to this need, I have included information here on many formulas that I have developed over the years. Some of these formulas are available commercially. All of them can be put together yourself by combining the nutrients recommended for each health care issue. Charts are also included in this chapter on the foods that contain the most important nutrients for women. For example, if you want to increase the level of vitamin C in your diet, the list on vitamin C-containing foods will help guide you as to which foods you need to emphasize.

Combining a high-nutrient diet with the careful use of nutritional supplements is often very helpful for women in the treatment and prevention of many female health problems.

How to Use Nutritional Supplements

This chapter includes formulas with specific recommendations for supplements, but I suggest that you start slowly. You may want to begin with as little as one-fourth of the listed dose, to see how well you tolerate the supplements. You can then increase your dose gradually until you find the level that works best for you.

I recommend that all supplements be taken with meals or at least with snacks. Very rarely, women experience nausea or diarrhea when beginning a supplement program. If this happens, your body is having difficulty tolerating a particular nutrient. In this case, stop all supplements. After a week you may want to begin your supplement intake again. Start with one supplement at a time until you discover which one is affecting you. You should probably eliminate that supplement from your program. Before taking any supplements, consult your physician or a nutritionist with specific questions about their use or possible side effects.

NUTRITIONAL SUPPLEMENTS FOR DAILY NEEDS

Vitamins and Minerals	Maximum Daily Dose
Vitamin A	5,000 IU*
Beta carotene (provitamin A)	10,000 IU
Vitamin B complex	
B_1 (thiamine)	25 mg*
B_2 (riboflavin)	25 mg
B_3 (niacinamide)	25 mg
B_5 (pantothenic acid)	50 mg
B_6 (pyridoxine HCl)	100 mg
B_{12} (cyanocobalamin)	100 mcg*
Folic acid	400 mcg

*IU=international units   mg=milligrams   mcg=micrograms

Biotin	300 mcg
Choline bitartrate	50 mg
Inositol	50 mg
PABA (para-aminobenzoic acid)	25 mg
Vitamin C	500 mg
Citrus bioflavonoids	200 mg
Rutin	25 mg
Vitamin D	400 IU
Vitamin E	100 IU
Calcium	250 mg
Magnesium	125 mg
Potassium	50 mg
Iron	18 mg
Chromium	100 mcg
Manganese	5 mg
Selenium	50 mcg
Zinc	15 mg
Copper	1 mg
Molybdenum	50 mcg
Iodine (from kelp)	100 mcg
Boron	1 mg
Silica	3 mg
Papain	50 mg
Betaine HCl	25 mg
Herbal base (from Dong quai, sarsaparilla, burdock root, false unicorn root, fennel, blessed thistle, red raspberry, peppermint, ginger root)	100 mg

Dosage: Take one-quarter to full amount of the above nutrients on a daily basis. Begin this formula with the lowest dose of each nutrient and increase the dose slowly and gradually, depending on how you are feeling.

NUTRITIONAL SUPPLEMENTS FOR PMS, MENSTRUAL CRAMPS, HYPOGLYCEMIA, AND HYPOTHYROIDISM

Vitamins and Minerals	Maximum Daily Dose
Beta carotene (provitamin A)	15,000 IU
Vitamin B complex	
B$_1$ (thiamine)	50 mg
B$_2$ (riboflavin)	50 mg
B$_3$ (niacinamide)	50 mg
B$_5$ (pantothenic acid)	50 mg
B$_6$ (pyridoxine HCl)	300 mcg
B$_{12}$ (cyanocobalamin)	50 mcg
Folic acid	200 mcg
Biotin	30 mcg
Choline bitartrate	500 mg
Inositol	500 mg
PABA (para-aminobenzoic acid)	50 mg
Vitamin C	1000 mg
Vitamin D	100 IU
Vitamin E	600 IU
Calcium (amino acid chelate)	150 mg
Magnesium	300 mg
Potassium	100 mg
Iron (amino acid chelate)	15 mg
Chromium	100 mcg
Manganese	10 mg
Selenium	25 mcg
Zinc	25 mg
Copper	0.5 mg
Iodine	150 mcg

Dosage: Take one-quarter to full amount of the above nutrients on a daily basis. Begin this formula with the lowest dose of each nutrient and increase the dose slowly and gradually to the recommended maximum, depending on how you are feeling.

HERBAL SUPPLEMENTS FOR PMS

Herbs (as capsules)	Maximum Daily Dose
Burdock	210 mg
Sarsaparilla	210 mg
Ginger	70 mg

Dosage: Take one to two capsules per day.

HERBAL SUPPLEMENTS FOR MENSTRUAL CRAMPS

Herbs (as tinctures)	Maximum Daily Dose
Ginger root	200 mg
White willow bark	200 mg
Chamomile	150 mg
Cramp bark	150 mg
Hops	150 mg
Sarsaparilla	150 mg

Mix dropperfuls of herbal tinctures in a glass of water. Begin at one quarter to one half of maximum dose. Increase to maximum recommended dose, if needed, slowly over several weeks. Find the dose that works best for you. You may divide this into a half dose that you use twice a day. Begin use of the herbs one week prior to the onset of your menstrual period.

NUTRITIONAL SUPPLEMENTS FOR FLUID RETENTION AND BLOATING

Vitamins, Minerals, and Herbs	Maximum Daily Dose
Vitamin B complex	
B_1 (thiamin)	15 mg
B_2 (riboflavin)	15 mg
B_3 (niacinamide)	15 mg
B_5 (pantothenic acid)	50 mg
B_6 (pyridoxine HCl)	100 mg
B_{12} (cyanocobalamin)	50 mcg
Folic Acid	400 mcg
Biotin	300 mcg
Choline bitartrate	25 mg
Inositol	25 mg
PABA (para-aminobenzoic acid)	25 mg
Vitamin C	250 mg
Citrus bioflavonoids	50 mg
Vitamin E	100 mg
Calcium	100 mg
Magnesium	50 mg
Potassium	50 mg
Iodine (from kelp)	150 mcg
Uva ursi	75 mg
Burdock root	75 mg
Sarsaparilla	75 mg
Dandelion root	50 mg
White willow bark	50 mg
Horsetail	50 mg
Corn silk	50 mg
Parsley	50 mg

Dosage: Take one to two tablets per day (up to maximum recommended daily dose).

NUTRITIONAL SUPPLEMENTS FOR CHRONIC FATIGUE SYNDROME, CANDIDA INFECTIONS, AND DEPRESSION

Vitamins and Minerals	Maximum Daily Dose
Beta carotene (provitamin A)	10,000 IU
Vitamin B complex	
B_1 (thiamine)	50 mg
B_2 (riboflavin)	75 mg
B_3 (niacinamide)	200 mg
B_5 (pantothenic acid)	200 mg
B_6 (pyridoxine HCl)	75 mg
B_{12} (cyanocobalamin)	100 mcg
Folic acid	400 mcg
Biotin	400 mcg
Choline bitartrate	700 mg
Inositol	500 mg
PABA (para-aminobenzoic acid)	50 mg
Vitamin C	2000 mg
Vitamin D	200 IU
Vitamin E	400 IU
Calcium aspartate	1200 mg
Magnesium aspartate	700 mg
Potassium aspartate	200 mg
Iron	18 mg
Chromium	150 mcg
Manganese	20 mg
Selenium	50 mcg
Zinc	15 mg
Copper	2 mg
Iodine (from kelp)	150 mcg

Dosage: Take one-quarter to full amount of the above nutrients on a daily basis. Begin this formula with the lowest dose of each nutrient and increase the dose slowly and gradually to the recommended maximum, depending on how you are feeling.

HERBAL SUPPLEMENTS FOR CHRONIC FATIGUE SYNDROME, CANDIDA INFECTIONS, AND DEPRESSION

Herbal Tinctures	Maximum Daily Dose
Ginkgo biloba	2 dropperfuls
Ginger root	2 dropperfuls
Burdock root	2 dropperfuls
Dandelion root	2 dropperfuls
Garlic	2 dropperfuls
Licorice root	1/2 dropperful

Dosage: Take one-quarter to full amount of the above nutrients on a daily basis. Begin this formula with the lowest dose of each nutrient and increase the dose slowly and gradually to the recommended maximum, depending on how you are feeling.

NUTRITIONAL SUPPLEMENTS FOR ANXIETY, PANIC, FOOD ADDICTIONS, ANXIETY COEXISTING WITH DEPRESSION, OR MITRAL VALVE PROLAPSE

Vitamins and Minerals	Maximum Daily Dose
Beta carotene (provitamin A)	25,000 IU
Vitamin B complex	
B_1 (thiamine)	50-100 mg
B_2 (riboflavin)	50-100 mg
B_3 (niacinamide)	50-100 mg

B_5 (pantothenic acid)	50-200 mg
B_6 (pyridoxine HCl)	50-200 mg
B_{12} (cyanocobalamin)	100 mcg
Folic acid	400 mcg
Biotin	400 mcg
Choline bitartrate	250-500 mg
Inositol	250-500 mg
PABA (para-aminobenzoic acid)	50-100 mg
Vitamin C	2000-5000 mg
Vitamin D	400 IU
Vitamin E	400-800 IU
Calcium aspartate	500-1000 mg
Magnesium aspartate	250-500 mg
Potassium aspartate	100-200 mg
Iron	81 mg
Chromium	150 mcg
Manganese	20 mg
Selenium	50 mcg
Zinc	15 mg
Copper	2 mg
Iodine (from kelp)	150 mcg

Dosage: Take one-quarter to full amount of the above nutrients on a daily basis. Begin this formula with the lowest dose of each nutrient and increase the dose slowly and gradually to the recommended maximum, depending on how you are feeling.

HERBAL-BASED NUTRITIONAL SUPPLEMENTS FOR ANXIETY, PANIC, FOOD ADDICTIONS, ANXIETY COEXISTING WITH DEPRESSION OR MITRAL VALVE PROLAPSE

(Note: Formula also contains vitamins and minerals in small amounts)

Vitamins, Minerals, and Herbs	Maximum Daily Dose
Vitamin B complex	
B_1 (thiamine)	1.5 mg
B_2 (riboflavin)	1.7 mg
B_3 (niacinamide)	20 mg
B_5 (pantothenic acid)	50 mg
B_6 (pyridoxine HCl)	5 mg
B_{12} (cyanocobalamin)	10 mcg
Folic acid	400 mcg
Biotin	300 mcg
Choline bitartrate	50 mg
Inositol	150 mg
PABA (para-aminobenzoic acid)	5 mg
Calcium	150 mg
Magnesium	150 mg
Passionflower	50 mg
Valerian root	50 mg
Chamomile	50 mg
Catnip	30 mg
Skullcap	25 mg
Celery	25 mg

Dosage: Take one-half to full amount of the above nutrients before going to bed at night or as needed (not to exceed twice the full dose in a four- to six-hour period) during times of stress.

NUTRITIONAL SUPPLEMENTS FOR ANEMIA

Vitamins and Minerals	Maximum Daily Dose
Iron	27 mg
Vitamin B complex	
B$_1$ (thiamine)	7.5 mg
B$_2$ (riboflavin)	7.5 mg
B$_6$ (pyridoxine HCl)	30 mg
B$_5$ (pantothenic acid)	50 mg
B$_3$ (niacinamide)	10 mg
B$_{12}$ (cyanocobalamin)	250 mcg
Folic acid	400 mcg
Biotin	100 mcg
Choline bitartrate	5 mg
Inositol	5 mg
PABA (para-aminobenzoic acid)	5 mg
Vitamin C	250 mg
Vitamin E (natural d-alpha)	30 IU
Zinc	1.5 mg
Copper	250 mcg
Betaine HCl	10 mg

Herbs	Maximum Daily Dose
Chlorophyll	2 dropperfuls
Yellow dock	2 dropperfuls
Pau d'arco	2 dropperfuls
Red clover	1 dropperful
Licorice root	1/2 dropperful

Dosage: Take one-quarter to full amount of the above nutrients on a daily basis. Begin this formula with the lowest dose of each nutrient and increase the dose slowly and gradually to the recommended maximum, depending on how you are feeling.

NUTRITIONAL SUPPLEMENTS FOR MENOPAUSE, HEAVY MENSTRUAL FLOW, FIBROID TUMORS, AND ENDOMETRIOSIS

Vitamins and Minerals	Maximum Daily Dose
Vitamin A	5000 IU
Beta carotene	5000 IU
Vitamin B complex	
B_1 (thiamine)	50 mg
B_2 (riboflavin)	50 mg
B_3 (niacinamide)	50 mg
B_5 (pantothenic acid)	50 mg
B_6 (pyridoxine HCI)	30 mg
B_{12} (cyanocobalamin)	50 mcg
Folic acid	400 mcg
Biotin	200 mcg
Choline bitartrate	50 mg
Inositol	50 mg
PABA (para-aminobenzoic acid)	50 mg
Vitamin C	1000–2000 mg
Bioflavonoids	800–2000 mg
Rutin	200 mg
Vitamin D	400 IU
Vitamin E (d-alpha tocopheryl acetate)	800–2000 IU
Calcium (calcium citrate)	1200 mg
Magnesium	320 mg
Potassium (potassium aspartate)	100 mg
Iron (ferrous fumarate)	27 mg
Chromium	100 mcg
Manganese	10 mg
Selenium	25 mcg
Zinc	15 mg
Copper	2 mg

Iodine (from kelp)	150 mcg
Bromelain	100 mg
Papain	65 mg
Boron	3 mg

Dosage: Women with mild to moderate menopause symptoms can use the formula at half strength. Women with severe symptoms should use the full strength.

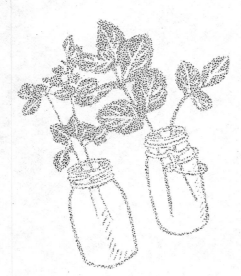

HERBAL SUPPLEMENTS FOR MENOPAUSE, HEAVY MENSTRUAL FLOW, FIBROID TUMORS, AND ENDOMETRIOSIS

Herbs (as capsules)	Maximum Daily Dose
Fennel	100–250 mg
Anise	100–250 mg
Blessed thistle	100–250 mg
False unicorn root	100–250 mg
Black cohosh	100–250 mg

Dosage: Take one to two capsules per day.

NUTRITIONAL SUPPLEMENTS FOR OSTEOPOROSIS

Vitamins, Minerals, and Herbs	Maximum Daily Dose
Vitamin B_6	10 mg
Vitamin B_{12}	25 mcg
Folic acid	200 mcg
Vitamin C	150 mg
Citrus bioflavonoids	250 mg
Vitamin D	400 IU

Vitamin K	25 mcg
Calcium	1000–1500 mg
Magnesium	400 mg
Manganese	10 mg
Zinc	7.5 mg
Copper	1 mg
Boron	1 mg
Silica	100 mcg
Vanadium	50 mcg
Sulfur	30 mcg
Betaine HCl	50 mg
Glucose polymers	50 mg
Fennel	100 mg
False unicorn root	100 mg
Black cohosh	100 mg
Blessed thistle	100 mg

Dosage: Take one-half to full amount of the above nutrients on a daily basis as needed.

NUTRITIONAL SUPPLEMENTS FOR HAIR, SKIN, AND NAILS

Vitamins, Minerals, and Herbs	Maximum Daily Dose
Vitamin A	5000 IU
Beta carotene	5000–50,000 IU
Vitamin B complex	
B_1 (thiamine)	15 mg
B_2 (riboflavin)	15 mg
B_3 (niacinamide)	40 mg
B_5 (pantothenic acid)	50 mg
B_6 (pyridoxine HCl)	20 mg
B_{12} (cyanocobalamin)	30 mcg

Folic acid	400 mcg
Biotin	400 mcg
Choline bitartrate	30 mg
Inositol	30 mg
PABA (para-aminobenzoic acid)	10 mg
Vitamin C	250 mg
Citrus bioflavonoids	50 mg
Vitamin D	200 IU
Vitamin E	100 IU
Calcium	150 mg
Magnesium	75 mg
Manganese	2 mg
Selenium	100 mcg
Zinc	15 mg
Copper	1 mg
Iodine (from kelp)	50 mcg
Flaxseed oil	250 mg
Horsetail	50 mg
Oat straw	25 mg
Burdock root	25 mg
Chamomile	25 mg
Ginger Root	25 mg
Ginkgo biloba	10 mg
Cayenne	25 mg
Egg albumin protein isolate (providing 100 mg of naturally occurring cystine and 50 mg of 1 methionine)	300 mg
GLA	20 mg

Dosage: Take one-quarter to full amount of the above nutrients on a daily basis. Increase dosage slowly if you do plan to use maximum daily dose (over several weeks).

Food Sources of Vitamins

FOOD SOURCES OF VITAMIN A

Vegetables
Carrots
Carrot juice
Collard greens
Dandelion greens
Green onions
Kale
Parsley
Spinach
Sweet potatoes
Turnip greens
Winter squash

Meat, Poultry, Seafood
Crab
Halibut
Liver—all types
Mackerel
Salmon
Swordfish

Fruits
Apricots
Avocados
Cantaloupe
Mangoes
Papaya
Peaches
Persimmons

FOOD SOURCES OF VITAMIN B COMPLEX (INCLUDING FOLIC ACID)

Vegetables and Legumes
Alfalfa
Artichokes
Asparagus
Beets
Broccoli
Brussels sprouts
Cabbage
Cauliflower
Corn
Garbanzo beans
Green beans
Green peas
Kale
Leeks
Lentils
Lima beans
Onions
Pinto beans
Romaine lettuce
Soybeans

Meat, Poultry, Seafood
Egg yolks*
Liver

Grains
Barley
Bran
Brown rice
Corn
Millet
Rice bran
Wheat
Wheat germ

Sweeteners
Blackstrap molasses

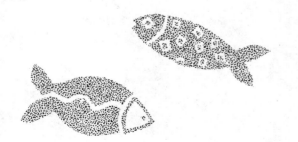

*Eggs and meat should be from organic range-fed stock, raised on pesticide-free food.

FOOD SOURCES OF VITAMIN B₆

Grains
Brown rice
Buckwheat flour
Rice bran
Rice polishings
Rye flour
Wheat germ
Whole wheat flour

Vegetables
Asparagus
Beet greens
Broccoli
Brussels sprouts
Cauliflower
Green peas
Leeks
Sweet potatoes

Meat, Poultry, Seafood
Chicken
Salmon
Shrimp
Tuna

Nuts and Seeds
Sunflower seeds

FOOD SOURCES OF VITAMIN B₁₂

Fish
Eggs
Liver

FOOD SOURCES OF BIOFLAVONOIDS

Alfalfa
Berries
Buckwheat
Cherries
Grapefruit

Grapes
Lemons
Limes
Oranges
Soybeans

FOOD SOURCES OF VITAMIN C

Fruits
Blackberries
Black currants
Cantaloupe
Elderberries
Grapefruit
Grapefruit juice
Guavas
Kiwi fruit
Mangoes
Orange juice
Oranges
Pineapple
Raspberries
Strawberries
Tangerines

Vegetables
Asparagus
Black-eyed peas
Broccoli
Brussels sprouts
Cabbage
Cauliflower
Collards
Green onions
Green peas
Kale
Kohlrabi
Parsley
Potatoes
Rutabaga
Sweet peppers
Sweet potatoes
Tomatoes
Turnips

Meat, Poultry, Seafood
Liver—all types
Pheasant
Quail
Salmon

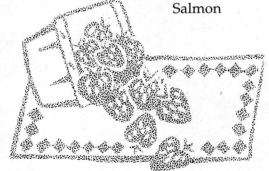

FOOD SOURCES OF VITAMIN E

Vegetables
Asparagus
Cucumber
Green peas
Kale

Nuts and Seeds
Almonds
Brazil nuts
Hazelnuts
Peanuts

Grains
Brown rice
Millet

Fruits
Mangoes

**Meat, Poultry,
Seafood**
Haddock
Herring
Lamb
Liver—all types
Mackerel

Oils
Corn oil
Peanut oil
Safflower oil
Sesame oil
Soybean oil
Wheat germ oil

FOOD SOURCES OF ESSENTIAL FATTY ACIDS

Corn oil
Flax oil
Grape oil
Pumpkin oil
Safflower oil

Sesame oil
Soybean oil
Sunflower oil
Walnut oil
Wheat germ oil

FOOD SOURCES OF CALCIUM

**Vegetables and
Legumes**
Artichokes
Beet greens
Black beans
Black-eyed peas
Broccoli
Brussels sprouts
Cabbage
Collards
Eggplant
Garbanzo beans
Green beans
Green onions
Kale
Kidney beans
Leeks
Lentils
Parsley
Parsnips
Pinto beans
Rutabaga
Soybeans
Spinach
Turnips
Watercress

**Meat, Poultry,
Seafood**
Abalone
Beef
Bluefish
Carp
Crab
Haddock
Herring
Lamb
Lobster
Oysters
Perch
Salmon
Shrimp
Venison

Fruits
Blackberries
Black currants
Boysenberries
Oranges
Pineapple juice
Prunes
Raisins
Rhubarb
Tangerine juice

Grains
Bran
Brown rice
Bulgar
Millet

FOOD SOURCES OF MAGNESIUM

Vegetables and Legumes
Artichokes
Black-eyed peas
Carrot juice
Corn
Green peas
Leeks
Lima beans
Okra
Parsnips
Potatoes
Soybean sprouts
Spinach
Squash
Yams

Fruits
Avocados
Bananas
Grapefruit juice
Papaya
Pineapple juice
Prunes
Raisins

Grains
Brown rice
Millet
Wild rice

Meat, Poultry, Seafood
Beef
Carp
Chicken
Clams
Cod
Crab
Duck
Haddock
Herring
Lamb
Mackerel
Oysters
Salmon
Shrimp
Snapper
Turkey

Nuts and Seeds
Almonds
Brazil nuts
Hazelnuts
Peanuts
Pistachios
Pumpkin seeds
Sesame seeds
Walnuts

FOOD SOURCES OF POTASSIUM

Vegetables and Legumes
Artichokes
Asparagus
Beets
Black-eyed peas
Brussels sprouts
Carrot juice
Cauliflower
Corn
Garbanzo beans
Green beans
Kidney beans
Leeks
Lentils
Lima beans
Navy beans
Okra
Parsnips
Peas
Pinto beans
Potatoes
Pumpkin
Soybean sprouts
Spinach
Squash
Yams

Meat, Poultry, Seafood
Bass
Beef
Carp
Catfish
Chicken
Cod
Duck
Eel
Flat fish
Haddock
Halibut
Herring
Lamb
Lobster
Mackerel
Oysters
Perch
Pike salmon
Scallops
Shrimp
Snapper
Trout
Turkey

Nuts and Seeds
Almonds
Brazil nuts
Chestnuts
Hazelnuts
Macadamia nuts
Peanuts
Pistachios
Pumpkin seeds
Sesame seeds
Sunflower seeds
Walnuts

FOOD SOURCES OF POTASSIUM, CONT.

Grains
Brown rice
Millet
Wild rice

Fruits
Apricots
Avocados
Bananas
Cantaloupe
Currants
Figs
Grapefruit juice
Orange juice
Papaya
Pineapple juice
Prunes
Raisins

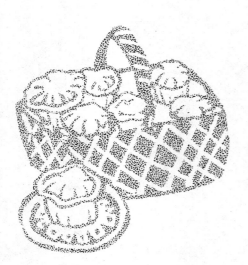

FOOD SOURCES OF IRON

Grains
Bran cereal
(All-bran)
Bran muffins
Millet, dry
Oat flakes
Pasta, whole wheat
Pumpernickel bread
Wheat germ

Legumes
Black beans
Black-eyed peas
Garbanzo beans
Kidney beans
Lentils
Lima beans
Pinto beans
Soybeans
Split peas
Tofu

Fruits
Apple juice
Avocados
Blackberries
Dates, dried
Figs
Prunes, dried
Prune juice
Raisins

Vegetables
Beets
Beet greens
Broccoli
Brussels sprouts
Corn
Dandelion greens
Green beans
Kale
Leeks
Spinach
Sweet potatoes
Swiss chard

Meat, Poultry, Seafood
Beef liver
Calves' liver
Chicken liver
Clams
Oysters
Sardines
Scallops
Trout

Nuts and Seeds
Almonds
Pecans
Pistachios
Sesame butter
Sesame seeds
Sunflower seeds

FOOD SOURCES OF ZINC

Grains
Barley
Brown rice
Buckwheat
Corn
Cornmeal
Millet
Oatmeal
Rice bran
Rye bread
Wheat berries
Wheat bran
Wheat germ
Whole wheat bread
Whole wheat flour

Fruits
Apples
Peaches

Meat, Poultry, Seafood
Chicken
Oysters

Vegetables and Legumes
Black-eyed peas
Cabbage
Carrots
Garbanzo beans
Green peas
Lentils
Lettuce
Lima beans
Onions
Soy flour
Soy meal
Soy protein

Part III

Food Preparation

CHAPTER 12

Food Handling and Preparation

A healthy diet starts with the careful handling and preparation of food. The finest basic ingredients can be turned into unhealthy dishes if the preparatory steps do not preserve the basic nutrient content of the food. This chapter recommends ways to store and prepare fruits, vegetables, seeds, nuts, and grains, as well as meat and fish. It also suggests the most healthful cooking techniques.

How to Select and Prepare Fruits and Vegetables

If at all possible buy organic or unsprayed fruits and vegetables. Try to avoid produce that has been sprayed with pesticides. Many people have become sick from ingesting heavily sprayed food. These chemicals accumulate in our bodies and weaken our immune systems. Many health food stores now carry unsprayed produce and, increasingly, so do the large grocery store chains. Call stores in your area and look for advertisements in your local newspapers for clean foods. If none are available locally, I recommend washing produce thoroughly in water and liquid soap to at least wash off the surface residues of pesticides. Nontoxic cleansing agents for produce are available in many health food stores.

Plant your own herbs, fruits, and vegetables. Produce grown from your own garden will be the ripest, freshest, and most delicious that you will ever taste. Luckily, millions of Americans take advantage of this bounty. Even if you live in areas with limited sunshine (Northern states), you can grow many delightful food plants in your own yard. Apartment dwellers can often grow a few foods, such as tomatoes, on their deck or herbs in a window box. Those who live in warmer states, obviously, can enjoy an extended growing season with a wider range of choices. Many of my friends have gardens as I do. This year I grew tomatoes, cucumbers, and mint. Last year, with more free time, I grew parsley, red and green peppers, and melons. After you have picked your own produce, be sure to avoid exposing it excessively to the sun. Letting fruits and vegetables sit in the sun after they've been picked causes them to wilt. Be sure to refrigerate them right away.

Buy seasonal produce. Each season brings a new bounty of fruits and vegetables. For example, melons, berries, peaches, and apricots appear in the summer, with apples and pears ripening into the fall. Buying seasonal produce will assure you a much wider variety of foods in your diet, which will increase and improve your range of nutrients. This is much more desirable than simply buying apples and oranges year-round which have either been cold-stored (and, therefore, not as fresh) or imported from a great distance. Some seasonal produce have the advantage of being locally grown. This produce will usually be fresher, more tender, and more flavorful than produce shipped from far away.

Avoid canned and frozen produce when possible. Many women buy processed fruits and vegetables even when fresh produce is available. This is due to the mistaken belief that preparing fresh produce is too time-consuming. Often the processed foods have lost valuable nutrients like vitamins B and C. They might also be laden with unhealthy levels of additives like sugar and salt. For example, canned vegetables often contain high levels of salt, while canned fruit is often packed in a sugary syrup. If you must buy processed produce, frozen food is a better bet than the canned varieties since additives are usually kept to a minimum. Buy canned fruit and vegetables either packed in water or their own juice.

Ideally, fruits and vegetables should either be eaten raw or with a minimum of preparation to preserve the nutrient content of the food. Simple, uncomplicated food preparation (which is the least time consuming) is actually best when preparing produce.

Eat the freshest produce possible. When shopping in a supermarket, avoid wilted-looking produce. This produce is either too old or has not been treated properly in the store. Many stores now use misting systems in the produce area, which keeps the fruits and vegetables better hydrated. The fruits and vegetables will look more attractive, last longer, and have a better texture if watered in the stores. Buy only a few days' supply of the most perishable items. It is better to shop for produce more frequently in smaller batches. This also helps to cut down on spoiled food and waste.

Store all produce properly. Be sure to store in your refrigerator all greens, peppers, parsley, and herbs immediately after purchase. While potatoes, winter squash, and onions store well in the refrigerator, they can also be stored in a cool area of your kitchen, such as a cupboard. This can be helpful for women with small refrigerators or limited storage area.

Tomatoes, avocados, and bananas are often not fully ripened when purchased in a supermarket. They can sit on your counter until they soften or change color. You might then want to store them in the refrigerator until you are ready to eat them. Summer fruits should be stored in the refrigerator immediately after purchase so that they do not spoil rapidly. Apples and pears can be kept in a bowl on your counter, but should be eaten quickly to avoid spoilage. Citrus fruits can also be kept on the counter in bowls for snacks. However, all fruits will keep best when refrigerated.

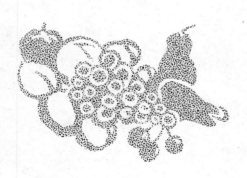

Serve fresh fruits and vegetables whole or cut into larger pieces. Eating fruits and vegetables whole or cut into large pieces tend to minimize the loss of their essential nutrients. This also helps to preserve flavor. Avoid peeling produce whenever possible (except to remove tough, discolored, or unsightly skin), since many nutrients are found just beneath the skin. For example, the white inner peel of citrus fruits contains high concentrations of bioflavonoids, which can help regulate female hormonal balance. Raw carrots, celery, jicama, broccoli, cauliflower, cabbage, spinach, tomatoes, cucumbers, mushrooms, and many other vegetables are delicious served whole or sliced into large pieces. They look lovely arranged in rows or circles on the plate and served with light dips or salad dressings. They are full of vitamins A and C, magnesium, calcium, and many other nutrients.

Use crisp and fresh ingredients to prepare salads. Lettuce should be well drained in a colander or on a paper towel. Rather than cutting leaf lettuce, gently tear the leaves by hand and toss them into the salad bowl. Add the dressing just before serving or serve several dressings on the side so that diners can select their own preference. Dark green vegetables such as romaine lettuce, endive, parsley, watercress, and red lettuce are more nutritious than iceberg lettuce. You can add a variety of tasty raw vegetables such as turnips, beets, carrots, cauliflower, water chestnuts, snow peaches, and jicama. Many of these vegetables contain high amounts of calcium, magnesium, iron, and other important nutrients. Cooked beans such as garbanzos (chick peas) and kidney beans are also excellent salad ingredients and are a fine source of protein.

Steaming helps to guard nutrients and flavor when cooking produce. When a recipe calls for cooking a vegetable to tenderize it, steaming is the best method of all. Produce can be steamed whole (as is often done with potatoes and corn) or cut into pieces for more rapid cooking. Simply place the food in a steamer, a basket that sits in the pot above boiling water. The food is cooked by the steam and doesn't touch the boiling water directly. After the water has boiled a few seconds, turn the flame low and place a lid on the pot to hold in the steam. Steamed foods have a much more interesting texture and taste than boiled food. Steaming takes no longer than preparing frozen vegetables or heating a TV dinner. Heavily boiled, baked, or sautéed produce are the most devoid of nutrients. These cooking techniques should be avoided.

Cook vegetables rapidly by oil-less stir-frying. This method can replace frying in many dishes and, thus, eliminate much fat. It can be done either in a frying pan or a wok. Instead of hot oil, use broth, bouillon, soy sauce, or water. Stir the foods into the hot liquid. This will cook them quickly and seal the juices into the food. Many vegetables contain enough natural sugar to brown using this method.

Store leftover produce carefully. Store leftover salad ingredients in a well-sealed plastic bag. This insures that the vegetables will remain fresh and crisp. Cooked fruits and vegetables to be reused for a future meal should be stored in air-tight plastic containers. Be sure to use all leftovers soon after the initial food preparation as they do not have a long shelf life.

How to Select and Store Seeds and Nuts

Buy nuts in their shells whenever possible. The old-fashioned habit of cracking nuts in their shell is actually the healthiest way to eat them. A variety of nuts and seeds are available preshelled in bins at health food stores and supermarkets. Unfortunately, the oils in nuts and seeds are very perishable and are partially rancid by the time you buy them. This is unfortunate since nuts and seeds are among our best sources of the essential fatty acid, linoleic acid, so necessary for female health. Some nuts and seeds, like walnuts, pumpkin seeds, and ground flax seeds are also good sources of the other essential fatty acid, linolenic acid. These fatty acids are light- and oxygen-sensitive and degrade rapidly, losing their healthful properties when exposed to air and light in store bins.

To preserve the essential fatty acids and other oils, refrigerate all seeds and nuts (and their oils). Unless nuts are in their shells, all seeds and nuts and their oils should be refrigerated immediately after purchase. This will help to preserve their freshness and avoid rancidity. Cold-pressed bottles of seed and nut oils should be refrigerated immediately after opening. Very perishable seed oils, like flax oil, are packed in opaque containers that keep out light and help to reduce their exposure to oxygen, so they should be refrigerated even before opening. Flax seed oil bottles are dated to ensure that they are used quickly to preserve their freshness. Flax seed oil can even be stored in the freezer, as can seeds and nuts, until you are ready to use them.

Eat seeds and nuts raw rather than roasted. Heat, like light and oxygen, can affect the integrity of the delicate seed and nut oils. Avoid eating roasted seeds and nuts whenever possible and select the raw versions instead. Also, avoid eating salted nuts and seeds. Many women find that they do not digest roasted and salted seeds well. The high-salt content of these foods can also worsen fluid retention and bloating in women with PMS or early menopausal symptoms.

Raw and unsalted seed and nut butters, especially almond and sesame seed butters, are now available in most health food stores. These are excellent, high-quality spreads which can be served on toast or crackers. They are much healthier and easier to digest than peanut butter. They are especially delicious when combined with fresh fruit preserves.

How to Select and Prepare Meat, Poultry, and Seafood

Buy range-fed meat and poultry if at all possible. Many meat and poultry producers keep the animals in close, cramped quarters. These animals are given hormones, antibiotics, and other chemicals to grow and fatten quickly. The meat is then often treated with chemicals as it is taken from the slaughterhouse to the supermarket so that it has a longer shelf life.

In contrast, range-fed meat and poultry are allowed to

roam, have a healthful and varied diet, and mature longer without the use of chemicals. I don't want dangerous chemical residues in my body and neither should you. I have also found range-fed meat to be more tender and flavorful. Range-fed meat and poultry are available at most health food stores and, increasingly, in supermarket chains.

Buy lean cuts of meat. Avoid prime meat, which is more expensive and marbled with fat, or fatty cuts like chuck steak. If you eat beef, use the leaner cuts of meat like flank steak and lean hamburger. Be sure to ask the butcher to trim all the extra fat off the meat or do this yourself at home. Poultry should have all the skin removed. This significantly decreases the calories as well as the fat content.

Try to eat fish at least once or twice a week. Certain fish are excellent sources of the essential fatty acid, linoleic acid. This includes salmon, trout, mackerel, and halibut. Linolenic acid is a precursor of the beneficial series-3 prostaglandin family of chemicals. These hormonelike chemicals help to lower your triglyceride levels and reduce the tendency for your blood cells to clump, which decreases the risk of strokes and heart attacks. Fish also contains many essential nutrients like iodine, which is essential for a healthy thyroid. It is low in calories and, for many people, is easier to digest than beef, pork, or lamb.

Try cooking meat, poultry, and fish by steaming, poaching, stewing, and simmering. Using those methods, meat can be cooked in water or vegetable juices rather than fat. Not only is meat tender and delicious when cooked this way, but the essential nutrients are preserved. Many traditional cuisines have employed steaming or poaching to cook fish. These methods are excellent for preparation of seafood as they preserve the delicate texture and flavor of the fish.

When roasting meat such as beef roast or poultry, place the meat on a rack. This enables the fat to drain. The meat should not sit in a pool of fat. This cooking technique helps to reduce the amount of saturated fat that you will be eating. The saturated fat, marbled in the flesh of meat or found under the skin of poultry, is one of the strong arguments against eating large quantities of these foods. These fats, when eaten in excess, increase the unhealthy LDL cholesterol levels in the body. These cholesterol levels have been implicated in cardiovascular disease, the major cause of death for American women and men.

When cooking meat in the oven, bake at low to moderate temperatures (325° to 375°F). Cooking temperature is very important. A low temperature allows meat to stay moist and tender and preserves more nutrients. The slow cooking of meat-containing dishes like soups and chilis in a crock pot is also preferred for preserving of nutrients.

Avoid deep-frying or pan-frying. These methods increase the fat content of meat. If you want to fry meat, try oil-less stir-frying. You can use a frying pan or wok. Instead of cooking with hot oil, use hot water, broth, bouillon, or soy sauce. The natural fat in meat will give it a delicious taste when it is cooked this way.

Avoid heavy, thick sauces and gravies. Many traditional American gravies and sauces are filled with oil, butter, cheese, and other high-stress ingredients. Examples include gravies made of flour and turkey or beef fat, or rich butter- and cream-based sauces often served on fine cuts of beef. Instead, serve the meat simply with a nonsalt seasoning mix, herbs, or no flavor enhancers at all. This will allow you to enjoy the delicious taste of the food itself.

Suggested Cooking Equipment

There are several pieces of equipment that can make your food preparation simple and easy:

Stainless steel steamer. Steaming is a highly recommended way to cook vegetables, fruits, and meat. No extra fat is used in the cooking process. The vitamin and mineral content of your food is retained in the cooking process. This is not the case in boiling, where essential nutrients are leached from the food.

Wok. A wok can be used to fry food with a minimum of oil. In fact, usually the fat in the meat or vegetables is all that is needed, along with a little water or broth for cooking. Delicious one-dish meals using meat, grains, and vegetables can be made in a few minutes.

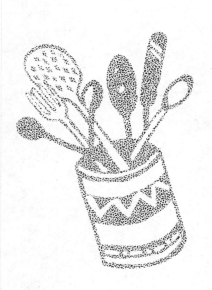

Juicer. A juicer is an indispensable item for many women. It allows fresh fruit and vegetables juices to be made as often as desired, on the spot, with all the essential nutrients preserved. A juicer also enables you to combine the types of fruits and vegetables that will enhance your health needs most. For example, women needing higher levels of beta carotene can combine carrots, spinach, and parsley in their juicer.

Blender. A blender can be used to make nondairy milk, smoothies, sauces, and purees of fruits and vegetables. A blender is relatively inexpensive and is a quick and easy way to prepare many high-nutrient foods. It is also excellent for women who need their food broken down because of dental or digestive problems.

Food processor. Salads, slaws, dough, and other foods requiring chopping, grating, and shredding can be made more rapidly using a food processor.

Stainless steel, glass, enamel, or iron pots and pans. Avoid using aluminum or copper cookware, as the metal can leach into your food. Acid foods interact with aluminum to form aluminum salts, which are toxic. Aluminum has been implicated in Alzheimer's disease, a disorder of the nervous system that impairs intellectual faculties and memory. When buying enamel cookware, be careful to buy a high-quality brand, as inferior enamel can chip away and expose the underlying metal. Cooking with iron pots, however, can actually provide useful supplemental iron for women who tend to be chronically iron-deficient due to heavy menstrual flow.

Shortcuts for Cooking and Storing Food

You can save a great deal of time by breaking up your tasks. Here are several methods that have worked for me over the years during extremely busy or stressful times:

Cook several meals at a time. For example, prepare two soups and a stew on the weekend. They can be frozen or refrigerated in meal-size containers without losing their nutritional value.

Speed up the cooking time of beans. Many women avoid cooking dried beans because it can take hours to boil and soften them. This can be discouraging if you are in a hurry. Here is a quick method:

Bring water to a boil (three cups of water for every cup of beans). Add the beans to the boiling water and cook for two minutes. Remove from the heat, partially cover the pan, and let beans cook for one hour. Go about your business or chores during this time as the beans continue cooking. After one hour, drain and rinse with cold water and then freeze.

When you are ready to use the beans for a meal, thaw them quickly under running water. Boil five cups of water in a pot for every cup of beans. Add the beans. Lower the heat and simmer for thirty to fifty minutes. The beans will be ready to use.

Prepare brown rice or grains in large quantities. Grains store for several days in the refrigerator in a jar or plastic container. They can be reheated and added to dishes when desired. Rice is best reheated by placing it over a double boiler or in a steamer and cooking it for three to five minutes. I do this often when my work schedule is extremely busy.

Freeze bread to keep it indefinitely. Make sure that the bread is stored in a plastic bag and sealed so that it is airtight. Slices of bread can be removed from the loaf and thawed gradually. They can also be placed in a toaster and warmed a few seconds.

Prepare hot cereal in a crock pot the night before. I do this all the time at home with oatmeal and other whole grain cereals. The cereals cook slowly overnight without my attention. They are absolutely delicious the following morning.

Trim and immediately wash leafy green vegetables and other salad makings after buying. They should be stored in plastic bags and refrigerated immediately. This will not only keep them fresher, but also will involve less work for you when you are ready to use them.

Store vegetable and chicken stock in the freezer indefinitely. Freeze stock in small amounts so that an entire pot of soup doesn't have to be defrosted for one meal and then refrozen. Try freezing it in ice cube trays.

CHAPTER 13

How to Substitute Recipes

*I*t is very important to learn how to adapt recipes so that they can be prepared with healthy ingredients. Most women have cookbooks and favorite recipes that produce delicious but unhealthy meals. Often these dishes are laden with ingredients such as caffeine, sugar, salt, alcohol, chocolate, dairy products, and fatty meats. Many of us were raised on food like this— main courses dripping in cream and butter or desserts that were rich and sugary. Obviously, dishes prepared in this way are not compatible with good health.

Luckily, you don't have to throw away your favorite cookbooks. Learning how to substitute healthy, nutritious foods in place of high-stress ingredients in recipes allows you to make your favorite foods without compromising your health. I have recommended this for years to my patients, who are pleased to find that they can still, have their cake and eat it too—but in a much healthier version.

Some women, however, choose to totally eliminate high-stress ingredients from a recipe. For example, when preparing a Chinese-style stir-fry dish, you can substitute tofu for beef and pork. The tofu has a chewy texture which many find appealing when used in combination with other ingredients. Alone it is bland, so it will take on the taste of the spices and sauces used in the recipe without disturbing the balance of flavors. For those women who wish to retain meat in their diet, skinless chicken can be used. You can also reduce the fat content of pasta dishes by eliminating the cheese. For instance, many women prepare pasta with tomato sauce, but forgo the parmesan cheese topping. Greek salad can be made without the feta cheese. Some of my patients even make pizza without cheese, layering tomato sauce and a variety of vegetables on the crust. In many cases, the high-stress ingredients are not necessary to make foods taste good.

If you want to retain a particular high-stress ingredient, you can usually reduce the amount of that ingredient, while still retaining the flavor and taste. Most of us have palates jaded by too much fat, salt, sugar, and other flavorings. In many dishes, we taste only the additives; we never really enjoy the delicious flavors of the foods themselves. During the last two decades, I have increasingly substituted low-stress ingredients in my own cooking. I find that I enjoy the subtle taste of the dishes much more. Also, I find that my health and vitality continue to improve with the deletion of high-stress ingredients from my food. The following information tells you how to substitute healthy ingredients in your own recipes. The substitutions are simple to make and should greatly benefit your health.

How to Substitute for Caffeinated Foods and Beverages

Drink decaffeinated coffee or tea as a transition beverage. If you cannot give up coffee, start by substituting water-processed decaffeinated coffee for the real thing. Then try to wean yourself from coffee altogether or try a coffee substitute. Some women may find the abrupt discontinuance of coffee too difficult because of withdrawal symptoms such as headaches. If this concerns you, decrease your total coffee intake gradually to only one or one-half cup per day. Use coffee substitutes for your other cups. This will help prevent withdrawal symptoms.

Drink grain-based coffee. Drinks like Pero, Postum, and Caffix actually taste somewhat similar to coffee, besides having its warmth and rich brown color. While nothing can exactly substitute for the flavor of coffee, many women find that these beverages provide a nice opener for the day when taken at breakfast. They are also handy to bring to work since they come in powdered form. Simply add water for a mid-morning or afternoon break.

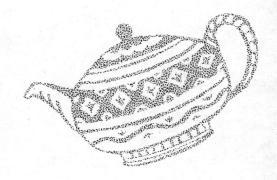

Drink herbal teas for energy and vitality. Many women who tend to be fatigued or stressed erroneously drink coffee as a pick-me-up to be able to function during the day. Drink ginger tea instead. It is a great herbal stimulant that won't wreck your health. To make ginger tea, grate a few teaspoons of fresh ginger root into a pot of hot water, boil, and steep. Serve with honey.

Substitute carob for chocolate. Chocolate is a common hidden source of caffeine. Luckily, carob provides a healthy alternative. Unsweetened carob tastes like chocolate but doesn't contain caffeine. It is a member of the legume family. Carob is also high in calcium. You can purchase it in chunks as a substitute for chocolate candy or as a powder for use in baking or drinks. Be careful, however, not to overindulge; carob, like chocolate, is high in calories and fat. Consider it a treat and an excellent cooking aid in small amounts only.

How to Substitute for Sugar

Substitute concentrated sweeteners. Americans tend to be addicted to sugar, consuming an average of 120 pounds per year. Most of us were raised on highly sugared soft drinks, candy, and rich pastries. I have found that as women decrease their sugar intake, most begin to enjoy the subtle flavors of the foods they eat even more. Concentrated sweeteners such as honey and maple syrup have a sweeter taste per quantity used than table sugar. Using these substitutes will allow you to decrease the actual amount of sugar you use in a recipe. If you use a concentrated sweetener in place of sugar in an ordinary recipe, reduce the liquid content in the recipe by one-fourth cup. If no liquid is used in the recipe, add 3 to 5 tablespoons of flour for each three-fourths cup of concentrated sweetener.

Substitute fruit for sugar in pastries. In making muffins and cookies, you may want to try deleting sugar altogether and adding extra fruits and nuts.

How to Substitute for Alcohol

Use low-alcohol or nonalcoholic products for cooking. Substitute low-alcohol or nonalcoholic wine or beer when cooking or preparing sauces and marinades. You will retain much of the flavor that alcohol imparts, and you will decrease the stress factor substantially.

Use low-alcohol or nonalcoholic beverages for making mixed drinks. Many people feel more comfortable at social functions holding a drink. And, too, they enjoy the fruity and frothy concoctions that are often whipped up at parties. Most of these drinks, though, can be made with fruit, sparkling mineral water, or a nonalcohol base. Don't feel shy to ask for your favorite drink prepared without alcohol when dining out at a restaurant or attending a social gathering. You might even start a trend.

How to Substitute for Dairy Products

Eliminate or decrease the amount of cow's milk cheese you use in food preparation and cooking. If you must use cow's milk cheese in cooking, decrease the amount in the recipe by three-fourths so that it becomes a flavoring or garnish rather than a major source of fat and protein. For example, use one teaspoon of parmesan cheese to top a casserole instead of one-half cup.

Use soy cheese in food preparation and cooking. Soy cheese is an excellent substitute for cow's milk cheese. It is lower in fat and salt, and the fat it does contain isn't saturated. In addition, many women are lactose intolerant and may have difficulty digesting cow's milk-based cheese. Health food stores offer many brands of soy cheese that come in a variety of flavors, such as mozzarella, cheddar, American, and jack. The quality of these products continues to improve. You can enjoy soy cheese as a perfect cheese substitute in sandwiches, salads, pizzas, lasagnas, and casseroles. In some recipes, you can replace cheese with soft tofu. I have done this often with lasagna, layering the lasagna noodles with tofu and topping it with melted soy cheese for a delicious dish. The tofu, which is bland, takes on the taste of the tomato sauce.

Replace milk and yogurt in recipes. For cow's milk, substitute potato milk, soy milk, nut milk, or grain milk. My personal favorite is a new nondairy milk, made from a potato base, called DariFree. It is easily digestible and particularly good for women with food allergies and digestive problems. It is creamy and sweet and tastes very similar to the best cow's milk, with none of the unhealthy side effects of dairy products. Even my 12-year-old daughter likes it. The potato-based milk is high in calcium and can be bought dry so that you can store it easily. Simply mix it with water and use it exactly as you would cow's milk for beverages, cooking, and baking. It will also be available soon in homogenized form in the dairy section of many supermarkets. DariFree, soy milk, rice milk, and nut milk are all available at most health food stores, as well as in some supermarkets. One benefit of soy milk is that it comes in many flavors. Many nondairy milks can be used for drinking, cooking, or baking.

For cow's milk-based yogurt, substitute soy yogurt. There are several excellent brands of soy yogurt currently available in the health food stores. They are available in plain, vanilla, and various fruit flavors. Another benefit is that these products tend to be cultured with live acidophilus, which is beneficial for the digestive tract. The taste is excellent and similar to cow's milk yogurt. I have found soy yogurt to be an excellent substitute in both cooking and baking.

Substitute flax oil for butter. Flax oil is the best substitute for butter that I've found. It is a rich, golden oil that looks and tastes quite a bit like butter. It is delicious on anything you'd normally top with butter—toast, rice, popcorn, steamed vegetables, or potatoes. Flax oil is extremely high in essential fatty acids—the type of fat that is very healthy for a woman's body. Essential fatty acids improve vitality, enhance circulation, and help promote healthy hormonal function. Flax oil is quite perishable, however, because it is sensitive to heat and light. For that reason, don't cook with it—cook the food first and add the flax oil before serving. Also, keep it refrigerated even before opening it. Because flax oil has so many health benefits, I highly recommend its use. You can find it in most health food stores.

How to Substitute for Red Meat and Poultry

Substitute beans, tofu, or seeds in recipes. You can usually modify recipes calling for hamburger or ground turkey by substituting tofu. For example, crumble up tofu to simulate the texture of hamburger and add it to recipes of enchiladas, tacos, chili, and ground beef casseroles. The tofu takes on the flavor of the sauce used in the dish and is indistinguishable from meat. I do this often when cooking at home.

When making salads that call for meat, such as chef's salad or Cobb salad, substitute kidney beans and garbanzo beans, along with sunflower seeds. These will provide the needed protein, yet are more easily digestible. You can also sprinkle sunflower seeds on top of casseroles to give it that extra zip, along with protein and essential fatty acids. When making stir-fries, substitute tofu, almonds, or sprouts for beef or chicken. Vegetable protein-based stir-fries taste delicious!

Use soy and wheat-based meat substitutes. For those women who want to prepare vegetarian food, yet still miss the taste and texture of meat, these products may provide the solution. Companies that produce these substitutes manufacture products that now taste astonishingly like sausage, hot dogs, hamburger, chicken, bologna, pepperoni, and other forms of meat. Be sure to check labels carefully as they can be high in fat and salt. For this reason, some of these meat-substitute products should be used sparingly.

How to Substitute for Wheat Flour

Use whole grain, nonwheat flour. For those women who are wheat-sensitive, substitute whole grain, nonwheat flours, like rice or barley flour. Whole grain flours are much higher in essential nutrients, such as vitamin B complex and many minerals. They are also higher in fiber. Rice flour makes excellent cookies, cakes, and other pastries. Barley flour is best used for pie crusts.

How to Substitute for Salt

Substitute potassium-based products for table salt (sodium chloride). Potassium-based products, such as Morton's Salt Substitute, are much healthier and will not aggravate heart disease or hypertension.

Use powdered seaweed such as kelp or nori to season vegetables, grains, and salads. Seaweed is a very healthy food, high in essential iodine and trace elements, and it tastes delicious.

Use herbs instead of salt for flavoring. The flavors of herbs are much more subtle and will help even the most jaded palate appreciate the taste of fresh fruits, vegetables, and meats.

Use liquid flavoring agents with advertised low-sodium content. Tamari, low-salt soy sauce, and Bragg's Liquid Aminos, a soybean-based flavoring agent, are delicious when used as salt substitutes in cooking. Add them to soups, casseroles, stir-fries, and other dishes at the end of the cooking process. You will find that you need only a small amount for intense flavoring.

Substitutes for Common High-Stress Ingredients

¾ cup sugar
    ½ cup honey
    ¼ cup molasses
    ½ cup maple syrup
    ½ oz barley malt
    1 cup apple butter
    2 cups apple juice

1 cup milk
    1 cup soy, potato, nut, or grain milk

1 cup yogurt
    1 cup soy yogurt

1 tablespoon butter
    1 tablespoon flax oil (must be used raw and unheated)

½ teaspoon salt
    1 tablespoon miso
    ½ teaspoon potassium chloride salt substitute
    ½ teaspoon Mrs. Dash or Spike
    ½ teaspoon herbs (basil, tarragon, oregano)

1½ cups cocoa
    1 cup powdered carob

1 square chocolate
    ¾ tablespoon powdered carob

1 tablespoon coffee
    1 tablespoon decaffeinated coffee
    1 tablespoon Pero, Postum, Caffix, or other grain-based coffee substitute

4 oz wine
    4 oz light wine

8 oz beer
    8 oz Near Beer

1 cup wheat flour	1 cup barley flour (pie crust)
	1 cup rice flour (cookies, cakes, breads)
1 cup meat	1 cup beans or tofu
	¼ cup seeds

Food Resources

Many women want to know what the best brands are of the commercially manufactured food products recommended in this book. The following products have received high marks for their good flavor from my patients. I also like them for their excellent nutrient quality. I use many of them when preparing the foods included this book's recipes. They are primarily available in natural food stores. As manufacturers are continually developing and introducing new products to address the changing market, be sure to enlist the help of your natural food store proprietor for further suggestions and recommendations.

Products	Manufacturers	Product Names
Nondairy milk	A&A Amazing Foods	DariFree
Soy cheese	Soyco, Soymage	Lite and Less
Soy cream cheese	Soya Kaas	Cream Cheese Style
Soy sour cream	Soymage	Sour Cream Style
Soy yogurt	White Wave, Nancy's	White Wave Dairyless
		Soy Yogurt
Soy frozen desserts	Turtle Mountain Inc.	Living Rightly
Guar gum (natural thickener)	Twin Laboratories	Guar Aid
Apple pectin (natural thickener)	Solgar	Apple Pectin Powder
Margarine (nonhydrogenated)	Spectrum	Spectrum Naturals Spread
Flax oil	Barlean's Organic Oils	Barlean's Flax Oil
Salt substitute	Bragg's Liquid Aminos	Live Food Products Inc
Wheat-free pasta	DeBoles	Angel Hair Pasta
		Rottini
		Artichoke Thin Spaghetti

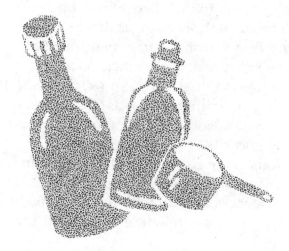

CHAPTER 14

Transition Easily and Effortlessly to a Healthier Diet

My patients often ask me, "How do I make the transition to a healthier diet?" It is a very important question, because a good strategy can make the difference between success and failure over the long term. While the information on foods to eat and foods to avoid serves as a base, most people find it difficult to make these changes in a gradual, practical way.

When first starting a treatment program, many of my patients have commented that their refrigerators and pantries are filled with food that they know they shouldn't eat. What should they do with these foods? Throw them away, give them away to friends and neighbors, or continue to buy and serve food they know they shouldn't be using?

Obviously, none of these solutions are in any woman's best interest. This chapter suggests practical guidelines that I have found to be most helpful with my patients. It also includes tips to enhance your enjoyment of a healthful and nutritious diet.

1. Keep your ultimate objective in mind when making all dietary changes. Most of you will be implementing these changes to enjoy better female and all-around general health. Many of you will also make changes to prevent health problems from occurring, so that you can enjoy an active and productive life. When eliminating foods from your diet that you are accustomed to but are harmful to your health, it is important to keep your long-term health goals in mind. This will make the process easier. Remember that you can enjoy excellent health as you get older. If you learn new techniques of wellness now, including good nutritional habits, your health can actually improve as you age.

2. Make all nutritional changes gradually. I have found in my medical practice that it takes anywhere from a month to two years to change one's dietary habits so that these changes feel comfortable and pleasurable (not just healthy). It is unrealistic to expect that you will throw away every high-stress food in your cupboard, although some women do make the transition that abruptly. It is important to find the pace that works for you.

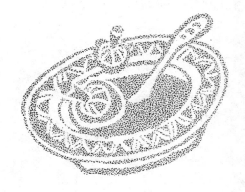

To make the transition to a healthier diet in an easy and nonstressful manner, I recommend you begin by making substitutions while continuing to eat the dishes that you are accustomed to. For example, substitute soy milk for cow's milk in your cereal or substitute a whole-grain, no-added-sugar cereal for a highly sugared, refined product. You might eliminate your daily cups of coffee by substituting herbal teas.

Rather than trying to make all the substitutions at once, select one or two foods that you would like to eliminate from your diet initially to improve your health. When you are comfortable with the changes you have made, consider making further modifications. Periodically review the list of foods to limit and foods to emphasize. Each time you review this list, select several more foods that you are willing to eliminate and foods to try. Review these lists as often as you choose, but try to do it on a regular basis. Every small change that you make in your diet can help your health tremendously.

As you eliminate high-stress foods from your diet, you might want to try cooking entirely new dishes using healthful ingredients. Eventually, you might want to restructure your meals entirely. Try the recipes and sample menus that I've provided in this book as models, and work with them to suit your tastes and the tastes of your family.

3. *Meals should be simple and easy to prepare.* Although elaborate and time-consuming meals are fun for parties or holidays, many women find that their day-to-day meals are best kept simple. Most women today lead busy, active lives and don't have much time to cook complicated meals. For that reason, I've kept my meal plans quick and easy to prepare, with the main emphasis on foods that are delicious and high in nutrition. For those women who often eat quick meals at fast-food restaurants or snack on commercial foods that are high in fat, sugar, and food additives, these simple meals offer a much healthier alternative.

Fortunately, nutritious foods can be just as delicious and convenient as less nutritious foods. Over the years, I have worked out many shortcuts for preparing high-quality food. Many of my patients have used these recipes and cooking tips to great advantage and can prepare a complete meal in 15 to 20 minutes (or even less).

4. *Don't feel guilty when you eat unhealthy foods.* We all have our favorite "sin" foods, like chocolate chip cookies, ice cream bars, and potato chips. Many of us turn to these foods during times of emotional stress since they are often associated with childhood comfort. Holidays make us face temptations that we don't have to deal with the rest of the year.

Don't become discouraged if you go off your diet for holidays, vacations, or just because your old food cravings become too strong. Everyone falls down at times. The successful person picks herself up and moves on. Just keep remembering your goals and reviewing the general guidelines I've outlined for you.

If you are using the guidelines in this book to help heal a specific female-related health problem, remember that healing occurs in a stepwise progression. It is never a straight line. Don't feel guilty if you go off your diet periodically if your general program is good. Great strides in healing can still be made with occasional desserts and junk food snacks.

5. Become your own best feedback system. If you are using this book to treat specific health problems, your own body will tell you when you have indulged too much in the wrong types of food. PMS symptoms or menstrual cramps may be worse during a month that you have eaten the wrong foods. You may find that you put on a few extra pounds due to bloating or fluid retention; menopausal flashes may occur more frequently. If your body gives you these messages, listen to them carefully. They are warning signals that you need to be stricter with your dietary choices. Conversely, when you are eating healthfully, symptoms have a tendency to fade away.

6. Nutritional changes can be fun. A positive attitude is very important when changing your diet. The entire process is delightful when you look upon it in a positive way.

The suggestions in this book offer a chance to taste new types of food and try out new recipes. Approach tasting these new foods as you would going to a new restaurant—with a sense of excitement. Many people consider dietary changes a punishment and think that once their health problems are better, they can return to their old eating habits. But it is these habits that often caused and worsened their symptoms in the first place, and are best left behind.

To maximize your enjoyment of your new food habits, emphasize the aesthetics of dining. A tablecloth, candles, and attractive serving dishes can dress up even simple fare. Highlight the color and texture of each food by using side dishes for serving. Try to serve foods with complementary colors. You will be widening your choice of nutrients as well as increasing visual appeal. (For example, red and yellow vegetables are high in vitamin A, while green vegetables are high in vitamin C.) This attention to aesthetics will increase your emotional gratification and sense of well-being.

7. Meals can still be family affairs. Eating healthy meals doesn't mean that you have to sit in a corner and eat by yourself. The nutritional suggestions in this book can be used with benefit by all members of your family and friends. Most of my patients find that their families enjoy sharing the new foods and feel healthier too.

Patients have reported to me that their husband's cholesterol levels and weight have plummeted following this program. Spouses' and children's allergy symptoms have cleared up, too. The health benefits can be dramatic for everyone.

Most dishes can be easily adapted to everyone's taste. If your children insist that life is empty without cheese or red meat, add some cheese and hamburger meat to one side of a casserole. Or prepare your side of a dish without the rich gravy the rest of your family likes or with more vegetables.

8. Eat the greatest possible variety of foods. Many women fall into the rut of eating the same foods day after day, going to the same shelves of the supermarket out of habit and convenience. There is safety in familiarity, in staying with a tried formula even if it adversely affects your health in the long run. Some women even have an initial fear or apprehension about trying new foods. Children certainly do. I've seen this over the years with my 12-year-old daughter and her friends.

For optimal health, it is best to be adventurous. Try new fruits and vegetables. Each season brings a bounty of produce different from the previous one. If you like almonds, try other nuts and seeds like sunflower, sesame, filberts, walnuts, and pecans. Don't always eat wheat as your source of grain. Cereals, breads, crackers, pastas, and even tortillas are now available in a variety of grains. By rotating your foods, you are assuring yourself the widest possible range of nutrients.

9. Eat heavier meals early in the day, lighter meals in the evening. Women who are weight conscious or have digestive problems may want to eat more lightly during the evening. Digesting food while you are asleep puts a large metabolic load on your entire system. Night is the time when your body repairs itself; it is unhealthy during this rest period to ask your body to continue to work. Weight also accumulates more easily when your main caloric intake is eaten after 7 p.m. Calories tend to be burned more efficiently during the earlier, more active part of the day. Thus, the calories from a large breakfast or lunch will be more thoroughly utilized by bedtime and not stored as fat.

10. Chew your food thoroughly. This is particularly important during the healing phase of any illness when you are trying to relieve the body of all significant stress. The first stage of digestion occurs in the mouth. Slow, thorough eating allows the food to be broken down before it reaches the stomach. Eating fast puts a strain on your digestive system. It will also cause you to eat more because you do not feel satiated until twenty minutes after you start eating. This can be a particular problem if weight gain or bloating are among your health issues.

Eating high-stress foods like beef, dairy products, and sugar products can cause fatigue or a sensation of heaviness. This is because so much energy is involved in the digestive process.

Take your time and enjoy your meals, however simple they are. Meal times are special times, to relax, to enjoy the company of friends or family, or to experience the pleasure of dining alone.

Part IV

Menus and Recipes

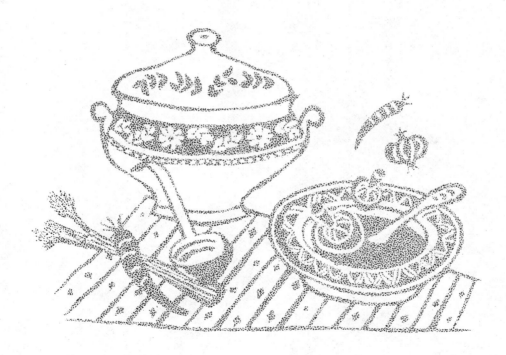

CHAPTER 15

Menus

Many women find the inclusion of menus in a nutritional program to be very helpful. For years, I have been giving my patients menus to help plan and organize their own meals. This chapter includes sample menus and breakfast, lunch, and dinner options for you to choose from. Use them as a guideline to develop your own meals. The recipes for quite a few of these dishes have been included in the recipe section that follows. Enjoy the meals and take pleasure in healthful dining.

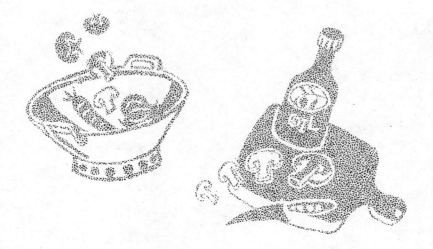

Breakfast Menus

Fruit smoothie
Raw pumpkin seeds
and sunflower seeds

Morning mock eggnog
Rice cereal with fruit and nuts

Flax shake
Rice cakes with strawberry preserves
Plain soy yogurt

Nondairy milk breakfast shake
Oat bran muffin
Applesauce

Instant flax cereal
Peppermint tea

Tofu cereal
Rose hip tea

Millet cereal with apricots
Fruit compote
Spring water

Oatmeal praline
Banana
Roasted grain beverage
(coffee substitute)

Oatmeal cereal and flax oil
Applesauce
Chamomile tea

Whole grain toast with peach preserves
Vanilla soy yogurt
Apple
Mint tea

Corn muffin with flax oil
Strawberries
Orange juice

Rice cakes
Raw sesame butter and
fruit preserves
Sliced grapefruit
Spring water

Brown rice cereal
Fresh carrot juice

All-bran cereal
Sliced strawberries
Soy milk

Wild rice pancakes
Peach slices
Peppermint tea

Pumpkin spice muffins
Banana
Ginger tea

Blueberry muffins
Orange juice
Raw almonds and sunflower seeds

Banana walnut muffins
Grapefruit slices
Roasted grain beverage
(coffee substitute)

Lunch and Dinner Meals

Soup Meals

Navy bean soup
Corn bread
Mixed green salad
Applesauce

Lentil soup
Mixed grain bread
Beet, radish, and cucumber salad
Dried figs

Vegetable and lentil soup
Steamed kale
Green beans
Dried apricots with almonds

Squash and potato soup
Steamed spinach
Broccoli with lemon juice
Dried pears

Onion soup
Coleslaw
Rye bread

Tomato soup
Kasha
Kidney beans

Split pea soup
Romaine salad
Whole wheat bread

Carrot soup
Calcium-rich vegetable salad
Bran muffins

Miso soup
Brown rice
Mixed green salad

Basic tofu soup
White rice
Steamed mustard greens

Black bean soup
Beet salad
Whole grain bread

Vegetable soup
Millet
Applesauce

Sandwich Meals

Tuna sandwich
Coleslaw
Apple

Vegetarian sandwich
Potato salad
Carrot and celery sticks

Avocado sandwich
Cheddar soy slices
Mixed green salad

Almond butter and
peach jam sandwich
Banana

Eggplant spread sandwich
Romaine salad

Sesame butter
and strawberry jam sandwich
Apple

Turkey sandwich
Potato salad

Falafel on pita bread
Lentil soup

Vegetable burger on a bun
Lettuce and tomato salad

Jack soy cheese sandwich with
avocado and tomato
Mixed green salad

Salad Meals

Buckwheat and potato salad
Vinaigrette dressing
Dried figs

Lentil salad
Wine vinegar, olive oil,
and basil dressing

Millet
Apple slices

Iron-rich fruit salad
Strawberry yogurt dressing
Banana walnut muffins

Beet salad
Vinaigrette dressing
Kidney beans

Tomato salad with green beans
Italian parmesan dressing
Baked potato with flax oil

Calcium-rich vegetable salad
Adzuki beans
Rye bread

Shrimp salad
Louie dressing
Sourdough bread

Spinach salad
Balsamic-honey dressing
Onion soup

Guacamole dip
Sliced carrots, red peppers,
and mushrooms
Corn tortillas

Tofu and wild rice salad
Fruit compote

Potato salad
Coleslaw
Sliced tomatoes
Bran muffins

Iron-rich vegetable salad
Vinaigrette dressing
Split pea soup

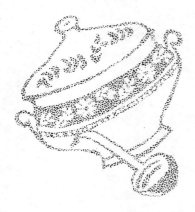

Main Courses and One-Dish Meals

Vegetarian Meals

Pasta with flax oil and garlic
Romaine salad
Two-bean dish
Mixed vegetable salad

Stuffed peppers with tomato sauce
Green beans and almonds
Steamed carrots

Hummus and tahini
Pita bread
Sliced carrots and cherry tomatoes

Rice and almond tabouli
Sliced tomatoes and cucumber

Mixed vegetable stir-fry
Brown rice

Kasha with zucchini and
tomato sauce
Vegetable soup
Rye bread

Tofu and almond stir-fry
Brown rice

Tofu and walnut rice
Hoisin sauce

Vegetarian tacos
Guacamole dip
Sliced carrots, red peppers,
mushrooms

Kasha Swiss melt
Applesauce

Seafood Meals

Poached salmon
Brown rice
Steamed carrots and peas

Broiled trout with dill
Baked potato with flax oil
Steamed artichoke

Broiled Tuna
Mixed green salad
Broccoli with lemon

Shrimp and millet stir-fry
Reduced-sodium soy sauce

Broiled sole with lemon
Sliced tomatoes and cucumber
Steamed red potatoes
Peas and carrots

Grilled halibut
Brown rice
Green beans and almonds
Coleslaw

Poached scallops
Mixed green salad

Grilled shrimp
Wild rice
Steamed broccoli

Grilled swordfish
Steamed red potatoes
Romaine salad

Poached flounder
Brown rice
Sliced tomatoes
Asparagus

Marinated fish
Mixed green salad

CHAPTER 16

Breakfast, Lunch, and Dinner Recipes

Breakfast

Contents:

Herbal Teas
Carob and Fruit Drinks
Nondairy Milk Beverages
Cereals
Pancakes and Muffins
Spreads

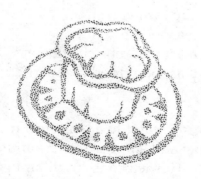

Herbal Teas

No wonder the English love teatime! There's nothing like curling up with a cup of hot herbal tea to relax and unwind, to soothe those raging moods, menstrual cramps, or digestive upsets. Energizing teas are miraculous, too. Imagine, a natural pick-me-up with no side effects.

PMS-Relief Tea   *Serves 2*

2 cups water   ½ teaspoon dandelion root
1½ teaspoons   1 to 2 teaspoons honey
   fresh ginger root, grated   (if desired)

Bring water to a boil. Add ginger and dandelion root and stir.
Turn heat to low and simmer for 15 minutes. Add sweetener if
desired.

   Ginger is a mild stimulant and helps relieve mood swings
and fatigue that are symptomatic of PMS. It can also relieve the
nausea that often accompanies menstrual cramps. Dandelion
root has a mild diuretic effect, which aids in controlling
PMS-related bloating and fluid retention. It is also rich in
essential minerals which help prevent PMS.

Menstrual Regulator Tea   *Serves 4*

4 cups water   1 teaspoon blackberry leaves
1 teaspoon rose hips   ¼ teaspoon orange peel
1 teaspoon hibiscus flowers   ¼ teaspoon lemon peel
1 teaspoon dried blueberries   2 teaspoons honey
                                                          (if desired)

Bring water to a boil. Add herbs to water and stir. Turn heat to
low and simmer for 15 minutes. Add sweetener if desired.

   This tea contains vitamin C and bioflavonoids which help
regulate menstrual flow and promote menstrual regularity.

Menopause Tea   *Serves 2*

2 cups water
2 teaspoons fennel
1 teaspoon honey (if desired)

Bring water to a boil. Add fennel to water and stir. Turn heat
to low and simmer for 15 minutes. Add sweetener if desired.
   Fennel is an excellent source of natural plant estrogens
(phytoestrogens). Fennel can be helpful for relieving
menopause symptoms like hot flashes, mood swings, and
fatigue. It also helps to relieve digestive gas.

Healthy Bladder Tea   *Serves 4*

4 cups water   1 teaspoon goldenseal
1 teaspoon parsley   ½ lemon, juiced
1 teaspoon fresh ginger root,   2 teaspoons honey
   grated   (if desired)
1 teaspoon uva ursi

Bring water to a boil. Add herbs and lemon to water and stir.
Turn heat to low and simmer for 15 minutes. Add lemon and
sweetener if desired.
   This tea promotes urinary tract health. Its mild diuretic
effect helps to promote the flow of urine. Goldenseal has an
antibiotic effect, which helps to prevent infections. Ginger
promotes good circulation to the bladder since it relaxes and
dilates the blood vessels.

Sleepytime Tea

Serves 4

4 cups water
1 teaspoon wild cherry

2 teaspoons chamomile
2 teaspoons honey
  (if desired)

Bring water to a boil. Add herbs to water and stir. Turn heat to low and simmer for 15 minutes. Add sweetener if desired.

    This mildly relaxing and sedative herbal tea is very useful for women with menopause-related sleeplessness.

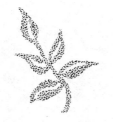

Energizing Herb Tea

Serves 2

2 cups water
2 teaspoons fresh ginger
  root, grated

1 teaspoon peppermint
  leaves
1 teaspoon honey (if desired)

Bring water to a boil. Add ginger and peppermint to water and stir. Turn heat to low and simmer for 15 minutes. Add sweetener if desired.

    This drink is an excellent coffee substitute. Both ginger and peppermint are stimulating herbs that can raise your energy level; ginger also helps relieve digestive problems, while peppermint quiets muscle spasms.

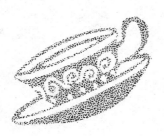

Relaxant Herb Tea

Serves 2

2 cups water
1 teaspoon peppermint
  leaves

1 teaspoon chamomile
  leaves
1 teaspoon honey (if desired)

Bring water to a boil. Add peppermint and chamomile leaves
to water and stir. Turn heat to low and simmer for 15 minutes.
Add sweetener if desired.

Peppermint and chamomile are both muscle relaxants and
antispasmodic herbs, so they can relieve pain and cramping
caused by menstrual cramps. They also help calm the mood,
which can be useful for women with PMS and menopause-
related mood swings.

Pain Relief Tea

Serves 2

2 cups water
1 teaspoon fresh ginger root,
  grated

1 teaspoon raspberry leaves
1 teaspoon honey (if desired)

Bring water to a boil. Add ginger and raspberry to water
and stir. Turn heat to low and simmer for 15 minutes. Add
sweetener if desired.

Ginger has both pain-relieving (analgesic) and antinausea
properties. Raspberry leaves have uterine relaxant properties
and help to relieve diarrhea. This is a helpful combination for
relief of menstrual cramps, fibroid and endometriosis
symptoms, and digestive complaints.

Beautiful Skin Tea

Serves 4

4 cups water
1 teaspoon gingko biloba
1 teaspoon cayenne pepper

2 teaspoons fresh ginger
  root, grated
2 teaspoons honey
  (if desired)

Bring water to a boil. Place herbs in water and stir. Turn heat to low and simmer for 15 minutes. Add sweetener if desired.

This tea helps to promote better blood circulation and oxygenation to the skin. It helps create rosy and youthful-looking skin. This tea also helps to warm the body and is useful for women who tend to have cold extremities or low body temperature and are sensitive to cold.

Arthritis Relief Tea

Serves 4

4 cups water
1 teaspoon white
  willow bark
3 teaspoons chamomile

½ lemon, juiced
2 to 4 teaspoons honey
  (if desired)

Bring water to a boil. Place herbs in water and stir. Turn heat to low and simmer for 15 minutes. Add lemon and sweetener, if desired.

White willow bark is an excellent anti-inflammatory herb which can help relieve joint pain. While its taste is bitter, it can be masked by the pleasant-tasting chamomile, which has been traditionally used to treat arthritis as well as relax muscle tension. Be careful, as white willow bark can occasionally cause gastric irritation in women with sensitive digestion.

Molasses Tea

Serves 1

1 cup warm water
2 teaspoons blackstrap molasses

Combine molasses and warm water. Stir thoroughly and serve. Molasses is an excellent source of calcium.

Ginger Tea

Serves 4

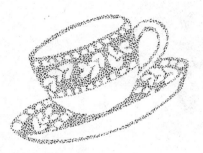

4 cups water
2 tablespoons ginger, grated
2 teaspoons honey (or other sweetener)

Add ginger to the water in a cooking pot. Bring to a boil and then turn heat to low. Steep for 15 or 20 minutes. Serve with honey or your favorite sweetener.

Ginger, without other herbs, makes a sweet, warming, and delicious tea.

Cold Relief Tea

Serves 4

4 cups water
2 teaspoons anise
2 teaspoons cinnamon

2 teaspoons honey
½ lemon, juiced

Bring water to a boil. Place remaining ingredients in water and stir. Turn heat to low and simmer for 15 minutes.

This sweet, spicy tea helps to relieve colds, coughs, and congestion.

Carob and Fruit Drinks

Here are some delicious and nutritious alternatives to hot chocolate and sodas. So many beverage options are available to quench our thirst and nourish our bodies. You must experience the zing of freshly made carrot and vegetable juice, tomato juice cocktails, fruit juice smoothies, or a blend of tropical fruit.

Hot Carob Drink

Makes 1 cup

1 cup hot water
2 tablespoons carob syrup

Fill cup with hot water. Add two tablespoons carob syrup (see recipe below). This drink looks and tastes like hot chocolate, but is far more healthy.

Carob Syrup

Makes 2 cups

1 cup water
¼ cup carob powder
1 cup honey

½ teaspoon vanilla
pinch salt

Combine water, honey, and carob powder in a cooking pot and bring to a rolling boil. Remove from heat and let cool. Add vanilla and salt. This syrup may be stored in the refrigerator.

Carrot Juice Cocktail #1

Serves 2

2 cups carrot juice
¼ cup beets

¼ cup fresh parsley
1 stalk celery

Juice beets, parsley, and celery. Mix with carrot juice and serve immediately.

Carrot Juice Cocktail #2

Serves 2

2 cups carrot juice
½ cucumber

2 beet tops
1 stalk celery

Juice cucumber, beet tops, and celery. Mix with carrot juice and serve right away.

Tomato Juice Cocktail

Serves 2

2 cups low-sodium tomato
  juice
½ cup carrot juice
¼ cup fresh parsley
¼ green pepper

8 spinach leaves
½ lemon, juiced
¼ teaspoon paprika
2 stalks celery

Juice parsley, green pepper, and spinach leaves. Combine with tomato and carrot juice. Add lemon juice and paprika, and stir well. Garnish with celery stalks and serve right away.

Fruit Shake

Serves 1

1 cup apple juice
½ cup nondairy milk
2 bananas

1 cup blackberries,
   blueberries, or strawberries

Combine apple juice, nondairy milk, bananas, and berries in a blender. Blend until smooth and serve.

Fruit Smoothie

Makes 2 to 3 cups

1 cup orange juice
2 bananas
¼ cup berries (blackberries, blueberries, raspberries,
   or strawberries)

Combine orange juice in a blender with bananas and your choice of berries. Blend until smooth and serve.

Cranberry Cocktail

Serves 2

2 cups cranberry juice
1 cup grape juice

½ lemon, juiced
2 teaspoons honey

Combine and serve.

Fruit Digestive Drink

Serves 2

¾ cup pineapple juice ½ cup orange juice
¾ cup papaya juice ¼ cup grapefruit juice

Combine in a blender and serve. Pineapple and papaya are
excellent sources of the digestive enzymes bromelain and
papain, and they taste delicious, too.

Apple-Lime Juice

Serves 2

2 cups apple juice
½ lime, juiced
½ to 1 teaspoon cinnamon

Combine in a blender and serve.

Nondairy Milk Beverages

Yes, Virginia, there is life after milk. I like the taste of nondairy
milk much better; and most of all, I like feeling better. For a
filling treat without milk's side effects, try a milkshake made
with flax oil, almonds, sesame seeds, or aloe.

Nondairy Milk Breakfast Shake

Serves 2

2 cups nondairy milk
2 ounces soft tofu
3 tablespoons flax oil
1 large banana

¾ cup berries
(strawberries,
boysenberries,
blueberries, or raspberries)

Combine all ingredients in a blender. Blend until smooth and serve.

Aloe Shake

Serves 2

1½ cups nondairy milk,
   plain or vanilla
3 tablespoons flax oil

¾ cup aloe, liquid
¾ cup frozen berries
1 large banana

Combine all ingredients in a blender. Blend until smooth and serve.

   Aloe is an herbal liquid that is extremely soothing and easy to digest. It is helpful and well tolerated by women with chronic fatigue and digestive problems.

Flax Shake #1

Serves 2

4 tablespoons raw flax seeds
2 bananas

¾ cup water
1 cup apple juice

Grind flax seeds to a powder using a coffee or seed grinder. Place powdered flax seeds in a blender. Add remaining ingredients and blend. Whole flax seed is high in essential fatty acids, calcium, magnesium, and potassium.

Flax Shake #2

Serves 2

4 tablespoons raw flax seeds
1 banana
1½ cups vanilla soy (or other) nondairy milk

Grind flax seeds to a powder using a coffee or seed grinder.
Place powdered flax seeds in a blender. Add remaining
ingredients and blend.

Whole flax seed is high in essential fatty acids, calcium,
magnesium, and potassium.

Soy Yogurt Shake #1

Serves 2

3 heaping tablespoons of soy
  yogurt (nondairy)
2 bananas
1 tablespoon of maple syrup
  or honey

1½ cups water
⅓ cup soy milk or other
  nondairy milk
2 tablespoons flax oil

Combine all ingredients in a blender and mix.

Soy Yogurt Shake #2

Serves 2

1 cup soy yogurt (or other
  nondairy yogurt)
1 cup orange juice
1 banana

2 tablespoons protein
  powder
1 tablespoon wheat germ

Combine all ingredients in a blender and mix.

Morning Mock Eggnog

Serves 1

1 cup water
1 banana
3 tablespoons flax oil

2 teaspoons honey or other
   sweetener
1 teaspoon nutmeg

Combine all ingredients in blender. Mix and serve for a rich, golden-yellow, eggnoglike drink.

Almond Milk

Serves 1

½ cup raw almonds
1 tablespoon honey or rice syrup
1 cup water

Combine almonds, honey, and ½ cup water in blender. Slowly add remaining water and blend until creamy. If you like a thinner milk, add 1 to 3 ounces more water.

Sesame Milk #1

Serves 1

3 tablespoons raw sesame
   butter or tahini
½ banana

½ cup apple juice
½ cup water
3 ice cubes

Combine all ingredients in blender for a delicious beverage.

Sesame Milk #2

Makes 2 cups

¾ cup apple juice
4 ice cubes
2 tablespoons tahini
  (sesame butter)
½ frozen banana

2 pitted dates
500 mg liquid or powdered
  calcium

Combine all ingredients in a blender and mix for a wonderful treat.

Cashew Milk

Makes 1¼ cups

½ cup cashews (or blanched almonds)
1 tablespoon honey or rice syrup
1 cup warm water

Combine cashews, honey, and ½ cup warm water in blender. Slowly add remaining water and blend until creamy. If you like a thinner milk, add 1 to 3 ounces more warm water.

Oat Milk

Makes 2 cups

½ cup rolled oats
2 cups water
⅓ banana
¼ teaspoon cinnamon

¼ cup apple juice
pinch of salt
250 mg liquid or powdered
  calcium (if desired)

Combine oats and hot water in a pot. Simmer in covered pot for 20 minutes. With remaining ingredients, whip in blender until smooth and creamy.

Cereals

Cereals are a staple in my house, made in minutes and served hot or cold to start the day, end the day, or even as a snack in between. I look forward to my morning cereal treat, loaded with fresh fruits and nuts, and the energy it gives me for hours.

Instant Flax Cereal

Serves 1

4 tablespoons raw flax seeds
scant ⅔ cup nondairy milk
  (soy or other base)

½ banana, sliced
1 to 2 teaspoons honey or
  other sweetener (to taste)

Grind raw flax seeds into a powder using a seed or coffee grinder. Place powder in a cereal bowl and slowly add the nondairy milk, stirring well until mixture is thickened to a texture similar to cream of rice or oatmeal. Top the cereal with sliced bananas. Add sweetener if desired. Eat right away, as flax seeds are sensitive to light, air, and temperature. This cereal should be eaten cold; do not cook this cereal. For variation, try adding nutmeg, allspice, cinnamon, or mace.

Tofu Cereal

Serves 2

4 ounces soft tofu
¼ cup nondairy milk
2 tablespoons flax oil
1 banana

1 apple
15 raw almonds
sweetener (if desired)

Combine all ingredients in a food processor. Blend until creamy. Pour into a bowl and serve. This is a nutritious cereal, high in natural plant estrogens, essential fatty acids, calcium, magnesium, and potassium. For variation, try adding mace, allspice, cinnamon, or nutmeg.

Praline Oatmeal

Serves 2

⅔ cup oats
1½ cups water
1 to 2 teaspoons maple syrup

1 tablespoon chopped raw
   pecans

Boil water in a pot. Stir in oats and return to a boil. Reduce heat to medium-low. Cook uncovered for 5 minutes, stirring occasionally. Remove from heat; let stand a few minutes. Stir in maple syrup. Top with pecans and serve.

Strawberries and Cream Oatmeal

Serves 2

⅔ cup oats
1½ cups water
4 ounces nondairy milk

1 to 2 teaspoons honey or
    other sweetener (optional)
¾ cup fresh strawberries

Boil water in a pot. Stir in oats and return to a boil. Reduce heat to medium-low. Cook uncovered for 5 minutes, stirring occasionally. Remove from heat; let stand a few minutes. Stir in nondairy milk and sweetener (if desired). Top with strawberries.

Mixed Berries Oatmeal

Serves 2

⅔ cup oats
1½ cups water
½ cup nondairy milk
1 to 2 teaspoons honey or
    other sweetener (optional)

½ cup blueberries
½ cup raspberries

Boil water in a pot. Stir in oats and return to a boil. Reduce heat to medium-low. Cook uncovered for 5 minutes, stirring occasionally. Remove from heat; let stand a few minutes. Stir in nondairy milk and sweetener. Top with berries.

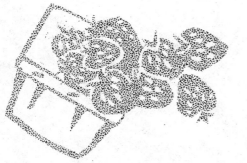

Oatmeal Cereal and Flax Seeds

Serves 2

⅔ cup oats
1½ cups water
2 tablespoons raw flax seeds,
  ground

¼ to ½ cup nondairy
  milk, vanilla
½ banana
2 teaspoons honey

Boil water in a pot. Stir in oats and return to a boil. Reduce heat to medium-low. Cook uncovered for 5 minutes, stirring occasionally. Remove from heat; let stand a few minutes. Stir in ground flax seeds, followed by nondairy milk and honey. Top with banana. Serve.

Oatmeal Cereal and Flax Oil

Serves 2

⅔ cup oats
1½ cups water

3 tablespoons flax oil
2 teaspoons maple syrup

Boil water in a pot. Stir in oats. Return mixture to a boil; reduce heat to medium-low. Cook uncovered for 5 minutes, stirring occasionally. Remove from heat and let stand a few minutes. Stir in flax oil and maple syrup. Serve.

All-Bran Cereal

Serves 1

⅛ cup All-Bran cereal
½ cup nondairy milk
⅛ cup ounce raisins

Combine cereal, nondairy milk, and raisins. (Strawberries may be added to increase vitamin C levels and, thereby, improve the iron absorption of this high-iron cereal.)

Brown Rice Cereal

Serves 2

2 cups cooked brown rice
½ cup vanilla nondairy
   milk or apple juice
2 tablespoons flax oil

10 raw almonds, chopped
2 teaspoons honey or
   other sweetener

Combine brown rice and nondairy milk or apple juice in a blender. Add almonds, flax oil, and honey, and serve.

Strawberries and Cream Rice Cereal

Serves 2

2 cups cooked brown rice
¾ cup nondairy milk,
   vanilla

½ cup strawberries
2 teaspoons honey or
   other sweetener

Combine brown rice and nondairy milk in a blender until smooth. Add strawberries and honey and serve.

Bananas and Cream Rice Cereal

Serves 2

2 cups cooked brown rice
¾ cup nondairy milk
1 medium banana, sliced

2 teaspoons honey or
   other sweetener

Combine brown rice and nondairy milk in a blender until smooth. Add bananas and honey and serve.

Rice Cereal with Fruit and Nuts

Serves 2

2 cups cooked brown rice
½ cup nondairy milk
½ apple, chopped
¼ cup raisins

8 almonds, chopped
4 walnuts, chopped
2 teaspoons honey or
   other sweetener

Combine brown rice and nondairy milk in a blender. Mix until smooth. Add apple, raisins, almonds, walnuts, and sweetener if desired, and serve.

Buckwheat Cereal with Blackberries

Serves 2

2 cups cooked buckwheat
   (kasha)
4 to 6 ounces nondairy milk

½ cup blackberries
2 teaspoons honey or
   other sweetener

Combine kasha and nondairy milk in a blender and mix well. Add blackberries and honey and serve.

Buckwheat Cereal with Bananas and Nuts

Serves 2

2 cups cooked buckwheat
   (kasha)
½ to ¾ cup apple juice
1 banana, sliced

8 almonds, chopped
2 teaspoons honey or
   other sweetener

Combine kasha and apple juice in a blender and mix well. Add bananas, almonds, and honey, and serve.

Buckwheat Cereal with Raisins and Almonds   *Serves 2*

2 cups cooked buckwheat   20 raisins
  (kasha)   12 almonds, chopped
¾ cup apple juice

Combine kasha and apple juice. Top with raisins and almonds
and serve.

Buckwheat Cereal with Filberts   *Serves 2*

2 cups cooked buckwheat
2 tablespoons maple syrup
12 filberts, chopped

Combine all ingredients in a bowl and serve.

Millet Cereal with Apricots   *Serves 2*

2 cups cooked millet   1 teaspoon raw sesame seeds
½ cup apple juice   1 tablespoon sunflower
5 dried apricots, sliced   seeds

Combine millet with apple juice and stir. Top with apricots,
sesame seeds, and sunflower seeds.

Millet Cereal with Peaches and Raspberries

Serves 2

2 cups cooked millet
1 cup nondairy milk
2 teaspoons honey or
   other sweetener

1 ripe peach, sliced
½ cup raspberries

Mix millet, nondairy milk, and honey. Garnish with raspberries and peach slices.

Millet Cereal with Prunes

Serves 2

2 cups cooked millet
¾ cup apple juice
6 prunes, chopped

Combine all ingredients in a bowl and serve.

Millet with Fruit and Nuts

Serves 2

2 cups cooked millet
¾ cup nondairy milk
2 teaspoons honey or
   other sweetener

½ apple, sliced
½ banana, sliced
8 almonds, chopped
6 filberts, chopped

Combine all ingredients in a bowl and serve.

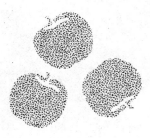

Millet Cereal with Molasses and Nuts

Serves 2

2 cups cooked millet
¾ cup apple juice

2 teaspoons molasses
10 almonds, chopped

Combine millet and apple juice. Add molasses and almonds. Stir gently and serve.

Pancakes and Muffins

Who wouldn't delight in the tantalizing aroma of freshly cooked hot pancakes, cornbread, or muffins? It's a wonderful way to welcome the weekend or any morning.

Brown Rice Pancakes

Serves 4

1 cup rice flour
¼ teaspoon salt
2 cups cooked brown rice
1 cup nondairy milk, vanilla

1 egg, separated
4 tablespoons flax oil
4 teaspoons maple syrup

Combine rice flour and salt in a large bowl; add rice. Beat nondairy milk and egg yolk together, then add to dry mixture. Beat egg white until stiff. Fold egg white into batter. Pour batter onto a lightly oiled hot griddle or frying pan. Cook on medium heat. Turn pancakes over when they begin to get crisp and brown. Top with flax oil and maple syrup and serve.

Wild Rice Pancakes

Serves 4

1 cup rice flour
¼ teaspoon salt
2 cups cooked wild rice
1 cup nondairy milk, vanilla
1 egg, separated

4 tablespoons flax oil
6 tablespoons strawberry or
   raspberry fruit purée or
   jam (no added sugar)

Combine rice flour and salt in a large bowl; add wild rice. Beat nondairy milk and egg yolk together and add to dry mixture. Beat egg white until stiff. Fold egg white into the batter. Pour batter onto a lightly oiled hot griddle or frying pan. Cook on medium heat. Turn pancakes over when they begin to get crisp and brown. Top with flax oil and fruit purée or jam. Serve.

Applesauce Oat Bran Muffins

Makes 8

2 cups oat bran
1 cup unbleached flour
3 teaspoons baking soda
2 teaspoons cinnamon
½ cup canola oil

½ cup applesauce
½ cup honey
½ cup apple juice
2 teaspoons vanilla

Preheat oven to 375°F. Combine all dry ingredients. In a separate bowl, combine all wet ingredients. Mix all ingredients together. Pour batter into oiled muffin tins ¾ full. Bake for 20 minutes or until center is cakelike. (Use the toothpick test: If an inserted toothpick comes out clean, your muffins are done.)

Orange Walnut Muffins

Makes 10

2 cups unbleached flour
6 packets Sweet N'Low
2½ teaspoons baking powder
¼ teaspoon baking soda
pinch of salt

¼ cup canola oil
2 eggs
1 cup orange juice
1 tablespoon lemon juice
½ cup walnuts, chopped

Preheat oven to 400°F. Combine all dry ingredients except walnuts. In a separate bowl, combine all wet ingredients. Combine all ingredients, mixing gently until batter is well blended and smooth. Add walnuts to the batter and mix well. Pour batter into oiled muffin tins ¾ full. Bake for 20 minutes or until center of muffin is caklelike in texture. (Use the toothpick test.)

Banana-Walnut Muffins

Makes 18

3 cups unbleached flour
3 teaspoons baking powder
3 teaspoons baking soda
¾ cup walnuts
1½ cup mashed bananas

1 cup nondairy milk, vanilla
½ cup canola oil
½ cup honey
2 teaspoons vanilla

Preheat oven to 375°F. Combine all dry ingredients. In a separate bowl, combine all wet ingredients. Mix all ingredients together until well blended. Pour batter into oiled muffin tins ¾ full. Bake for 25 minutes or until center is cakelike. (Use the toothpick test.)

Pumpkin Spice Muffins

Makes 16

3 cups unbleached flour
3 teaspoons baking soda
½ cup raisins
2 teaspoons cinnamon
½ teaspoon ground allspice

½ teaspoon ground
  coriander
2 cups cooked pumpkin
1 cup apple juice
½ cup canola oil

Preheat oven to 375°F. Combine all dry ingredients. In a separate bowl, combine all wet ingredients. Mix all ingredients together. Pour batter into oiled muffin tins ¾ full. Bake for 30 minutes or until golden brown.

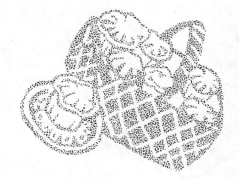

Soy Cornbread

Makes 1 loaf

2 cups cornmeal
½ cup soy flour
1 teaspoon baking powder
½ teaspoon baking soda
¼ teaspoon sea salt

1 egg, beaten
2 cups nondairy milk
3 tablespoons honey
2 tablespoons canola oil

Preheat oven to 425°F. Combine cornmeal, soy flour, baking powder, baking soda, and sea salt in a mixing bowl. Combine egg, nondairy milk, honey, and canola oil in a separate bowl. Mix all ingredients together and blend until batter is smooth. Pour into an oiled pan and bake for 30 to 35 minutes or until knife comes out clean upon testing.

Spreads

Creamy nut butters and fresh fruit toppings transform toast into a luxurious and filling treat. Try these spreads on pancakes and waffles, too.

Tofu and Sesame Butter Spread
Makes 1½ cups

½ cup tofu, drained
1 cup raw sesame butter
1 to 2 tablespoons honey

Blend all ingredients in a blender or food processor.

Sesame-Almond Butter
Makes 1½ cups

¼ cup soft tofu, drained
¼ cup raw sesame butter
6 tablespoons raw almond butter
⅛ cup honey

Combine all ingredients in a blender.

Apple-Spice Butter
Makes 2 cups

1 pound apples, peeled,
   quartered, and cored
¼ to ½ cup water
½ teaspoon cinnamon
⅛ teaspoon cloves
¼ teaspoon ginger
1 to 2 tablespoons honey

Cook apples in butter until soft. Add water and cook for 5 to 10 minutes. Add spices and honey to pan. Stir to mix. Cool. Blend in blender or food processor until smooth.

Instant Peach Spread

Makes 3 cups

3 cups canned peach slices (with liquid removed)
¼ cup honey
1½ teaspoon guar gum

Mix peaches and honey in a food processor until smooth. Add guar gum and blend. You can use this spread on pancakes, waffles, or even nondairy frozen desserts. It will keep in the refrigerator for up to 2 weeks.

Instant Mixed Berry Spread

Makes 3 cups

1¼ cup blueberries, fresh
   or frozen
1¼ cup blackberries, fresh
   or frozen

½ cup honey
1 teaspoon apple pectin

Combine berries and honey in a food processor and blend well. Add pectin and mix well again. This spread can be stored in the refrigerator for up to 2 weeks. Use on toast, rolls, pancakes, or waffles.

Fresh Applesauce

Serves 2

2 large apples
½ cup fresh apple juice

½ teaspoon cinnamon
⅛ teaspoon ginger

Cut apples into quarters; remove cores. Combine all ingredients in a food processor. Blend until smooth. Note: for a smooth texture, peel may be removed.

Raspberry Spread   *Makes 2 cups*

1¼ cup raspberries, fresh or frozen
¼ cup honey
⅓ cup water

Combine ingredients in a food processor and blend well. You
can use this spread with pancakes, waffles, and muffins.

Strawberry Spread   *Makes 2 cups*

2 cups strawberries,   ⅓ cup water
   fresh or frozen   1 to 2 tablespoons honey
2 tablespoons peach jam

Combine ingredients in a food processor and blend until
smooth. Try this spread on pancakes, waffles, and muffins.

Lunch and Dinner

Contents:

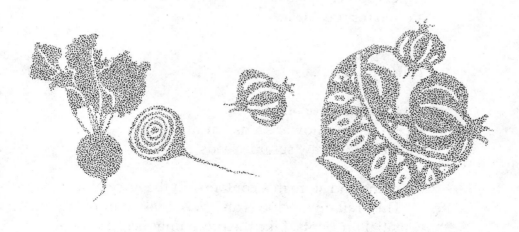

Snacks and Hors d'oeuvres

Hors d'oeuvres are not only deliciously appetizing, they help stave off hunger while dinner is cooking. It is better to eat often in small amounts. You won't feel guilty eating these healthy snacks. Popcorn is one of my favorites, especially with a variety of international species and flavors.

Trail Mix #1   *Makes 1½ cups*

½ cup raw pumpkin seeds, unsalted
½ cup raw sunflower seeds, unsalted
½ cup raisins

Combine and store in a container in the refrigerator.

    This trail mix recipe is very high in iron, calcium, magnesium, essential fatty acids, and other important nutrients. I use it as a snack to replace stressful and unhealthy sugar-based sweets and chocolate. It is a great mix to take on trips, and I eat it often for breakfast.

Trail Mix #2   *Makes 1 cup*

½ cup dried apricots
½ cup raw sunflower seeds, unsalted
2 tablespoons raw sesame seeds

Combine and store in a container in the refrigerator.

    This trail mix recipe is also very high in iron and other essential nutrients. Like the preceding recipe, I use it as a snack to replace stressful and unhealthy sugar-based sweets and chocolate.

Rice Cakes with Nut Butter and Jam
Serves 2

4 rice cakes, unsalted
2 tablespoons raw almond
   butter

2 tablespoons fruit preserves
   (no added sugar)

Spread almond butter and fruit preserves on rice cakes for a quick snack. Herbal tea makes a good accompaniment.

Rice Cakes with Tuna Fish
Serves 2

4 rice cakes, unsalted
4 ounces tuna fish
2 teaspoons low-calorie mayonnaise

Combine tuna and mayonnaise and spread on rice cakes. This is an excellent high-protein, high-carbohydrate snack.

Apple with Almond Butter
Serves 2 to 4

1 apple, sliced
1 tablespoon raw almond butter

Spread almond butter on apple slices.

Banana with Sesame Butter
Serves 2

1 banana, halved
1 tablespoon raw sesame butter

Spread sesame butter on each half of a ripe banana.

Spicy Pepper Dip

Makes 1 cup

1 cup (8 ounces) soy cream
   cheese
3 tablespoons sweet
   red pepper, chopped
2 cloves garlic, minced

3 tablespoons lime juice
¼ to ½ teaspoon
   Tabasco sauce
¼ teaspoon Worcestershire
   sauce

Combine in a food processor. Blend until smooth. Serve with raw, sliced mushrooms, green onions, and carrots.

Low-Fat Green Onion and Horseradish Dip

Makes 1 cup

½ cup green onion,
   finely minced
1¼ teaspoons horseradish,
   grated

1 teaspoon Dijon mustard
2 tablespoons low-calorie
   mayonnaise

Combine all ingredients in blender. Blend until smooth. This is an excellent dip for vegetables such as carrots, red pepper, and broccoli, as well as a tasty dip for shrimp and crab.

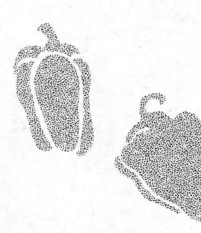

Southwestern Chunky Bean Dip

Makes 2½ cups

1 cup cooked kidney beans
1 cup vegetarian
  refried beans
½ small red onion,
  chopped
1 medium clove garlic,
  minced

1 teaspoon Anaheim pepper,
  finely minced
⅛ teaspoon cumin
½ teaspoon oregano
½ teaspoon Bragg's Liquid
  Aminos
1 ripe tomato

Combine all ingredients except tomato in food processor and blend until smooth. Transfer dip to a serving dish, add chopped tomato, and gently stir. This dip is excellent with no-oil tortilla chips, fresh vegetables, and guacamole.

Sherried White Bean Dip

Makes 1 cup

2 cups cooked white beans
1 shallot, minced
½ teaspoon parsley,
  minced
2 tablespoons sherry (or nonalcoholic brand sherry)

¼ teaspoon Bragg's Liquid
  Aminos
2 teaspoons canola oil

Combine all ingredients in a blender and blend until smooth. Use as a spread on French bread, crackers, toast, melba toast, and rye bread.

Italian White Bean Dip

Makes 1 cup

2 cups cooked white beans
¼ red onion, finely
　chopped
1 clove garlic, minced
¼ teaspoon parsley,
　minced

½ teaspoon Italian
　seasoning
⅛ teaspoon sea salt
1 tablespoon olive oil
1½ teaspoons Balsamic
　vinegar

Combine all ingredients in a blender and blend until smooth. Use as a spread on French bread, crackers, toast, melba toast, and rye bread.

Sherried Black Bean Dip

Makes 1⅓ cups

2 cups cooked black beans
1 shallot, minced
½ teaspoon parsley,
　minced
½ teaspoon chives

2 teaspoons canola oil
¼ teaspoon Bragg's
　Liquid Aminos
2 tablespoons Madeira wine

Combine all ingredients in a blender and blend until smooth. Use as a spread on French bread, crackers, toast, melba toast, and rye bread.

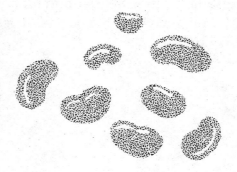

Spinach Dip

Makes 3 cups

1 pound soft tofu
4 tablespoons low-calorie
   mayonnaise
1 cup spinach, chopped
½ teaspoon nutmeg

1 teaspoon low-sodium
   soy sauce
1 teaspoon sherry
½ teaspoon guar gum

Combine all ingredients in a food processor and blend well.

Spicy Tomato Dip

Makes 2 cups

8 ounces soft tofu
2 tablespoons low-calorie
   mayonnaise

¾ cup ketchup (Hain or
   other high-quality brand)
¼ teaspoon tabasco sauce

Combine all ingredients in a blender and blend until smooth.
This is an excellent sauce for falafels, shrimp, and crab.

Baked Tomato Bruschetta

Serves 4

8 slices crusty sourdough or Italian bread
3 tablespoons olive oil
2 cloves garlic, minced
3 large tomatoes, cut into chunks

¾ cup fresh basil, finely chopped and loosely packed
4 tablespoons soy parmesan

Preheat oven to 450°F. Toast bread until lightly brown. Drizzle with 1½ tablespoons olive oil and garlic. Heat remainder of olive oil in a frying pan over medium heat. Then turn to high and quickly sauté tomatoes and basil for a minute. Spread on toasted bread. Place on baking sheet and bake for 5 minutes. Sprinkle soy parmesan cheese on top after removing tomato bread from oven, and serve immediately.

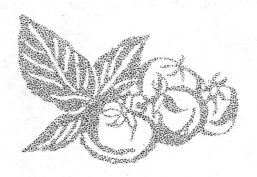

Eggplant Bruschetta

1 small eggplant, finely diced
3 tablespoons olive oil
1 small red onion, diced
1 clove garlic, minced
6 medium mushrooms,
   chopped
10 black olives, sliced
2 tomatoes, diced

2 teaspoons basil
2 teaspoons oregano
½ teaspoon parsley
¼ teaspoon rosemary
½ teaspoon sea salt
1 teaspoon sherry vinegar
8 slices crusty Italian bread

Steam eggplant for 5 to 6 minutes or until soft. In a pan, heat olive oil and sauté onion, garlic, mushrooms, and olives until vegetables begin to soften and the onion and garlic turn slightly golden brown. Add tomatoes to the pan and continue to cook for another minute, stirring well. Add basil, oregano, rosemary, sea salt, parsley, and eggplant. Continue to stir. Add sherry vinegar. Toast bread in oven or toaster until golden brown. Remove from oven and top with eggplant mix.

Stuffed Mushrooms

Serves 4

12 extra large mushrooms
1 tablespoon canola oil
1 small red onion,
   finely diced
¾ cup fresh spinach,
   finely shredded

¼ cup firm tofu,
   finely crumbled
¼ teaspoon sea salt
¼ cup bread crumbs
2 tablespoons sherry (or nonalcoholic brand sherry)

Preheat oven to 350°F. Clean mushrooms and remove stems. Dice stems and place to one side. Pour canola oil in frying pan. Combine stems, red onion, spinach (be sure spinach is well washed), tofu, and sea salt and place in frying pan. Cook until vegetables are soft or golden brown. Add bread crumbs, mix well, and add sherry. Continue to mix for a minute. Remove from heat. Stuff mushroom caps with filling, place them on a baking sheet, and cook in oven for a few minutes.

Marinated Mung Bean Sprouts #1

Serves 4

4 cups mung bean sprouts
2½ tablespoons seasoned
   rice vinegar

1⅓ teaspoons sake
2 teaspoons low-sodium
   soy sauce

Combine all ingredients in a mixing bowl and blend well. Let sit for 10 minutes and serve.

Marinated Mung Bean Sprouts #2 *Serves 4*

4 cups mung bean sprouts
3 tablespoons seasoned
   rice vinegar
2 teaspoons low-sodium
   soy sauce

¼ teaspoon ginger powder
¼ teaspoon garlic powder

Combine all ingredients in a mixing bowl and blend well. Let sit for 10 minutes and serve.

Babaganouj

2 medium eggplants
½ cup tahini
1 tablespoon flax oil
3 cloves garlic

1 teaspoon salt
pinch cayenne pepper
pinch black pepper
juice of ½ lemon

Preheat oven to 375°F. Prick eggplants with a fork about six times each. Place directly on oven rack and bake approximately 45 minutes, until soft and squishy. Cut the top of each eggplant off and discard. Cut each in half lenghthwise and scoop out the pulp. Place pulp in blender, add remaining ingredients and blend until smooth.

Popcorn and Flax Oil *Serves 2*

½ cup popcorn
2 tablespoons flax oil
½ teaspoon salt substitute

Air-pop the popcorn into a large bowl. Sprinkle with flax oil and salt substitute.

Spicy Popcorn

Serves 2

4 cups air-popped popcorn
1 teaspoon olive oil
¾ teaspoon Bragg's
   Liquid Aminos

½ teaspoon paprika
¼ teaspoon garlic powder

Add olive oil and Bragg's slowly to popcorn, drizzling over the kernels. Mix popcorn well. Add paprika and garlic powder and mix well. Bragg's may be applied to popcorn with spray container.

Mexican Popcorn

Serves 2

4 cups air-popped popcorn
1 teaspoon olive oil
½ teaspoon chili powder
¼ teaspoon paprika

⅛ teaspoon cumin
¼ teaspoon oregano
1/16 to ⅛ teaspoon sea salt

Drizzle olive oil over popcorn and mix well. Add chili powder, paprika, cumin, oregano, and sea salt and mix well.

Oriental Popcorn

Serves 2

4 cups air-popped popcorn
1 teaspoon canola oil
¾ teaspoon low-sodium
   soy sauce

¼ teaspoon ginger powder
¼ teaspoon garlic powder

Drizzle canola oil and soy sauce over popcorn and mix well. Add ginger and garlic powder and mix well.

Soups

Soup is multifaceted. As a starter, a light soup can turn any meal into elegant dining. A heartier soup can be a delightful meal in itself, especially when served with warm, chunky bread and a salad.

Vegetable Soup

Serves 6

4 tomatoes, diced
1 onion, chopped
1 turnip, chopped
½ leek, chopped
1 cup green peas
2 carrots, chopped
8 mushrooms, sliced

1 bay leaf
½ tablespoon thyme
½ tablespoon oregano
1 to 1½ quarts water
½ teaspoon salt substitute
¼ bunch parsley, chopped

Place all ingredients except parsley in a pot. Cover with water. Bring to a boil, then turn heat to low. Cook for 45 minutes. Pour the soup into individual serving dishes. Garnish with chopped parsley.

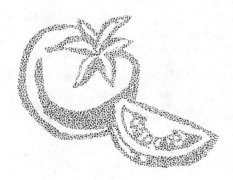

Potassium Broth

Serves 8 to 10

8 fresh tomatoes, medium-sized
4 cups water
1 cup carrots, sliced
1 cup broccoli, sliced
1 cup squash (zucchini or summer squash), sliced
½ cup mushrooms, sliced

½ cup celery, chopped
1 onion, diced
2 garlic cloves, minced
2 tablespoons fresh parsley, chopped
¼ to 1 teaspoon fresh or dried basil (to taste)

Liquefy tomatoes in a blender. Combine all ingredients in soup pot and bring to a boil for 30 minutes. Turn heat to low and simmer for another 30 minutes. Strain and serve.

Vegetable Lentil Soup

Serves 4 to 6

3 tomatoes, diced
½ cup lentils
½ onion, chopped
1 turnip, chopped
½ leek, chopped
½ cup green peas
2 carrots, chopped

8 mushrooms, sliced
½ tablespoon fennel
1 bay leaf
1½ quarts water
½ teaspoon salt substitute
¼ bunch parsley, chopped

Wash lentils. Place all ingredients except parsley in a pot. Bring to a boil, then turn heat to low. Cook for 2 hours. Pour the soup into individual serving dishes. Garnish with chopped parsley.

Split Pea Soup   *Serves 4*

1 cup dried split peas
½ onion, chopped
1 small carrot, sliced

4 cups water
¼ to ½ teaspoon sea salt
  or salt substitute

Wash peas. Place peas, onion, and carrot in a pot. Add water.
Bring to a boil, then turn heat to low and cover pot. Cook for
45 minutes. Add sea salt and continue to cook until peas are
soft. Soup may be cooled and then puréed in a blender if you
prefer a creamy texture.

Black Bean Soup   *Serves 4*

1 cup black beans
4 cups water
1 onion, chopped
2 cloves garlic, diced

1 carrot, diced
1 potato, diced
2 teaspoons tamari

Wash and drain black beans. Place beans and water in
a pot, cover, and bring to a boil. Turn heat to low and
cook approximately 2 hours or until beans are tender.
(Presoaking beans in water overnight will lessen cooking
time; alternatively, precooked, canned beans may be used.)
Add remaining ingredients. Bring to a boil, then turn heat to
low, and cook until beans and vegetables are done.

Lentil Soup

Serves 4

1 cup dried lentils	4 to 6 cups water
½ onion, chopped	1 teaspoon brown rice miso
½ cup carrots, chopped	

Wash lentils. Place all ingredients in a pot. Bring to a boil, then turn heat to low, cover pot, and simmer for 45 minutes or until lentils are soft. Vary the amount of water depending upon the desired thickness of soup.

Carrot Soup

Serves 4

4 cups carrots, peeled and sliced	1½ tablespoons ginger root, grated
1¼ cups onions, diced	1½ cups nondairy milk, vanilla
½ cup sweet red pepper	
4 cups vegetable broth	

Combine carrots, onions, red peppers, vegetable broth, and ginger in a large pot. Cook for 30 minutes or until carrots are tender. Strain vegetables and reserve the broth. Purée vegetables in a food processor. Blend together and purée broth, nondairy milk, and vegetables. Return soup to cooking pot. Cook on low for five minutes. Serve.

Squash and Potato Soup

Serves 6

4 summer squash
   (crookneck), sliced
1 potato, diced
1 onion, chopped
3 cups water

½ teaspoon low-salt soy
   sauce (or salt substitute)
1 teaspoon thyme
⅛ bunch parsley, minced

Steam squash, potato, and onion; place vegetables in a pot. Add water and cook on low heat in covered pot for 15 minutes. Add low-salt soy sauce and thyme and continue cooking for another 15 minutes, until vegetables are soft. After cooking, purée vegetables in blender. Garnish with minced parsley.

Tofu Soup

Serves 8

1 onion
2 large carrots
1 cup tofu, diced

1 to 1½ quarts vegetable
   stock
¼ to 1 teaspoon basil

Chop vegetables into bite-sized pieces. Place them in uncovered pot. Add tofu and vegetable stock. Bring to a boil. Turn heat to low, cover pot, and let soup cook until vegetables are soft. Add basil and sea salt to taste.

Variations: Add any combination of the ingredients. All have high nutritional value for women and will add flavor to the soup.

Miso Soup   *Serves 4*

4½ cups water
2 carrots, sliced
1 onion, sliced
¼ head cabbage, chopped

4 tablespoons red miso
2 tablespoons scallions or
   parsley, minced

Heat ½ cup water in pot. Add carrots and onion and cook
for 7 minutes. Add another ½ cup water and the cabbage; cook
for 5 more minutes. Add the remainder of the water, cover pot,
and bring to a boil. Turn heat to low and simmer for 15
minutes. Cream the miso with a little cooking water, add to
pot, and remove from heat. Sprinkle with scallions or parsley.
Serve.

Gazpacho   *Serves 4*

2 cups low-salt tomato juice
1 cup peeled tomatoes,
   chopped
½ cup green peppers,
   chopped
½ cup cucumbers, diced
¼ cup onions, chopped
2 tablespoons parsley,
   chopped

1 tablespoon chives, minced
2 garlic cloves, minced
2 tablespoons tarragon
   vinegar
2 tablespoons olive oil
½ teaspoon sea salt
¼ teaspoon black pepper
½ teaspoon Worcestershire
   sauce

Combine all ingredients in a stainless steel or glass container.
Chill overnight.

Onion Soup   *Serves 4*

2 pounds yellow onions,
   thinly sliced
3 cloves garlic, minced
3 tablespoons canola oil
6 ounces Near Beer

2½ cups vegetable broth
1 teaspoon Bragg's Liquid
   Aminos
1 tablespoon soy parmesan
   cheese

Sauté onions and garlic in the canola oil until lightly brown, stirring as needed. Add Near Beer, vegetable broth, and Bragg's Liquid Aminos; simmer for 35 minutes. Add croutons (see below) to the soup before serving. Sprinkle with soy parmesan cheese.

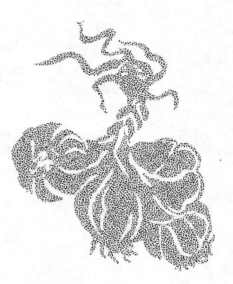

Croutons

2 slices sourdough bread*
2 tablespoons canola oil

Cut bread into cubes. Place in skillet with canola oil and cook, stirring frequently, until golden brown.

* If sourdough bread is not available, another crusty bread like rye may be used.

Wild Rice Soup

Serves 6

4 tablespoons canola oil
1 yellow onion, chopped
1 cup mushrooms, sliced
3 cups nondairy milk
1 tablespoon rice flour (or unbleached flour)

4 cups cooked wild rice
2 cups water
1 teaspoon nutmeg
1½ teaspoon sea salt
2 tablespoons marsala wine
2 teaspoons guar gum

Heat canola oil in a soup pot or wok on medium. Add onion and mushrooms and cook until lightly browned. Combine with nondiary milk. Add remaining ingredients, except guar gum, and mix well. Cook for 10 minutes. Sprinkle guar gum slowly over the soup and blend well. Continue to cook on low for an additional 20 minutes.

Butternut Squash-Carrot Soup

Serves 8 to 10

1 butternut squash, approximately 2 pounds
2 carrots, chopped
1 tablespoon canola oil
1 onion, chopped

4 cups nondairy milk
1 teaspoon mace
2 tablespoons maple syrup
2 cups cooked wild rice

Peel and chop butternut squash into ¾-inch cubes. Steam carrots and squash for 20 minutes or until soft. Heat canola oil in a skillet on high and sauté onion quickly for 2 to 3 minutes or until golden brown. Combine squash, carrots, nondairy milk, mace, and maple syrup in a food processor; blend until smooth. Transfer soup mixture to a pot and add onions and wild rice. Cook for 5 minutes and serve.

Creamy Pea Soup   *Serves 4*

2½ cups cooked peas,
   fresh or frozen
1 cup vegetable broth
1½ cups nondairy milk
½ teaspoon parsley,
   minced

¼ teaspoon dried mint
   leaves
⅛ teaspoon sea salt
½ teaspoon guar gum

Purée peas in a food processor until smooth. Add remaining ingredients and mix well. Soup may be heated in a cooking pot.

Salads

In just a few minutes, you can dazzle the eye and the taste buds with the colorful array of fresh fruit or vegetables aesthetically arranged on a serving plate. Try mixing various colors and shapes like an artist preparing the palate.

Mixed Green Salad   *Serves 4 to 6*

1 head green or red leaf
   lettuce
1 large tomato, cut into
   wedges
½ cucumber, sliced

2 green onions, chopped
1 carrot, sliced
4 radishes, sliced
1 avocado, sliced
¼ cup sunflower seeds

Combine all ingredients in a large salad bowl. Serve with Ranch Dressing.*

*Note: See Salad Dressing recipes for all dressings suggested in this section.

Romaine Salad #1

Serves 4

1 head romaine lettuce
½ head red cabbage,
  chopped

4 radishes, sliced
1 small carrot, grated

Combine all ingredients in a bowl. Serve with Italian Parmesan Dressing.

Romaine Salad #2

Serves 4

1 head romaine lettuce
¼ red onion, chopped
4 mushrooms, sliced

Combine all ingredients in a large salad bowl. Serve with Vinaigrette Dressing.

Escarole-Butter Lettuce Salad

Serves 2

½ head butter lettuce
3 cups escarole, chopped (very loosely packed)
1 small tomato, sliced

Combine butter lettuce and escarole in a salad bowl. Add tomato slices. Serve with Terry's Rice Vinegar Vinaigrette Dressing.

Radicchio, Endive, and Escarole Salad

Serves 4

½ head endive
8 leaves radicchio
¼ head escarole

On each salad plate, arrange 4 leaves of endive, cover with radicchio, and top with escarole. Serve with Terry's Rice Vinegar Vinaigrette Dressing. For variation, add mushrooms, wild rice, red peppers, or sliced tomatoes.

Tomato Salad with Green Beans

Serves 4

1 pound green beans
1 tomato, chopped
3 teaspoons green onions, minced
1 garlic clove, minced
¼ teaspoon black pepper
1 teaspoon oregano

Steam green beans for 6 minutes. Texture should be crisp. Combine all ingredients in a large salad bowl. Serve with Italian Parmesan or Vinaigrette Dressing.

Watercress Salad

Serves 4

2 bunches watercress
¾ cup fresh bean sprouts
2 teaspoons scallions, finely chopped
½ tablespoon sunflower seeds
Vinaigrette dressing (to taste)

Wash watercress. Remove the large stems and place the rest in a bowl. Add bean sprouts and scallions. Toss salad. Add sunflower seeds and Vinaigrette Dressing and toss again.

Calcium-Rich Vegetable Salad

Serves 6

1 head romaine lettuce
1 avocado, sliced
¾ cup turnips, sliced
¾ cup celery, diced

¾ cup green onions, sliced
¾ cup watercress
¾ cup carrots, grated

Combine all ingredients in a large salad bowl and toss lightly.
Serve with Low-Calorie French Dressing.

Iron-Rich Vegetable Salad

Serves 4 to 6

1 head green or red leaf
  lettuce
1 large tomato, cut into
  wedges
6 mushrooms, sliced

2 green onions, chopped
¾ cup cooked
  kidney beans
1 avocado, sliced
¼ cup raw sunflower seeds

Combine all ingredients in a large salad bowl. Serve with
Vinaigrette Dressing.

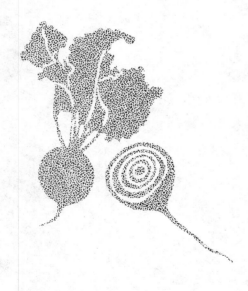

Beet Salad

Serves 4

3 medium steamed beets,
  diced
1 medium red onion,
  chopped

½ bunch parsley, chopped
½ red pepper, diced
¼ cup sunflower seeds

Combine all ingredients in a large salad bowl. Serve with
Vinaigrette Dressing.

Spinach Salad

1 bunch spinach, chopped
½ small red onion,
  chopped
⅓ cup red pepper, diced

½ cup mung bean sprouts
¼ cup firm tofu, diced
¼ raw sunflower seeds

Combine vegetables, tofu, and sunflower seeds in a large salad bowl and mix well. Serve with Balsamic-Honey Dressing.

Potato Salad

Serves 6

8 medium red potatoes
1 cup celery, chopped
½ cup parsley, finely
  chopped
½ cup green pepper,
  chopped

½ cup sweet raw onions,
  chopped
4 tablespoons mayonnaise
1 to 2 teaspoons Dijon
  mustard
1 teaspoon honey or other
  sweetener

Steam potatoes for approximately 45 minutes. Cool and cube. Combine celery, parsley, pepper, and onion with potatoes, and mix thoroughly. Add mayonnaise, Dijon mustard, and sweetener; mix until dry ingredients thoroughly combine with others.

Parmesan Potato Salad

Serves 4

2 pounds small red potatoes
½ small red onion,
    chopped
12 black olives, sliced
2 teaspoons capers
¼ cup olive oil

1 to 2 tablespoons cider
    vinegar
1 teaspoon Dijon mustard
3 teaspoons soy parmesan
    cheese

Steam potatoes for 35 minutes or until cooked. Cool and cut into eighths. In a large bowl, combine potatoes, onions, olives, and capers; add olive oil, cider vinegar, and mustard and blend gently. Top with soy parmesan cheese and mix again.

Coleslaw

Serves 4

½ teaspoon celery seeds
½ teaspoon poppy seeds
½ teaspoon dill seeds
2 cups red cabbage, finely
    shredded

1½ cups green cabbage,
    finely shredded

Crush or grind the seeds and add to shredded cabbage. Serve with your favorite dressing, such as oil and vinegar or honey dressing. The herbs used are high in calcium, magnesium, and iron.

Shrimp Salad with Louie Dressing

Serves 4

½ head iceberg lettuce
½ head romaine lettuce
8 mushrooms, sliced
½ small red onion, in rings

1 hard-boiled egg, quartered
1 avocado, quartered
½ pound shrimp, cooked
 and deveined

Combine lettuce, mushrooms, and onion. Top with egg, avocado, and shrimp; mix well. Serve with Louie Dressing.

Shrimp Salad

Serves 4

¾ pound bay shrimp
¾ cup green peas
3 tablespoons low-calorie
 mayonnaise
½ teaspoon tarragon,
 to taste

8 leaves butter lettuce
1 small cucumber, sliced
1 medium tomato, sliced
½ red pepper, thinly sliced
½ avocado, thinly sliced

Combine bay shrimp, peas, mayonnaise, and tarragon. Mound on lettuce leaves. Arrange the remaining vegetables around the plate.

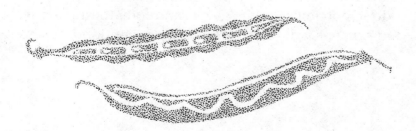

Cold Pasta and Shrimp Salad

Serves 4

3 cups fusilli pasta
10 shrimp, medium
12 spears asparagus,
  steamed and chopped
1 small red onion, diced
2 green onions, chopped

1 red pepper, chopped
6 mushrooms, sliced
16 black olives, sliced
6 tablespoons parsley,
  minced

Cook fusilli pasta for 12 minutes or until al dente. Place pasta to one side. Devein shrimp and remove the shells; cook in boiling water for one minute and 15 seconds. Remove shrimp from stove and place in cold water until chilled. Cut each shrimp into 3 pieces. Combine all ingredients in a large bowl. Serve with Vinaigrette Dressing.

Guacamole Dip #1

Serves 4

2 ripe avocados
2 tablespoons lemon juice
1 green onion, diced
1 garlic clove, minced

1 tomato, chopped
2 carrots, sliced
1 red pepper, sliced
4 large mushrooms, sliced

Peel avocados. Place them in a bowl and mash with a fork. Add lemon juice, onion, garlic, and tomato, stirring well. Chill and serve as a dip for the carrots, peppers, and mushrooms.

Guacamole Dip #2

Serves 2

2 ripe avocados
2 tablespoons low-salt salsa
2 carrots, sliced

1 red pepper, sliced
4 large mushrooms, sliced

Peel the avocados. Place in a bowl and mash with a fork. Add the salsa and mix well. Use as a dip with carrots, peppers, and mushrooms.

Iron-Rich Fruit Salad

Serves 4

½ cantaloupe, cubed
16 strawberries
2 bananas, sliced

1 cup pineapple, cubed
½ cup raisins
4 lettuce leaves

Combine fruit in a large serving bowl. Mix gently. Spoon mixture onto lettuce leaves. Serve with Strawberry Yogurt Dressing.

Carrot-Raisin Salad

Serves 2

3 carrots
½ cup raisins

1 tablespoon mayonnaise
1 tablespoon cider vinegar

Peel and grate carrots. Mix carrots and raisins with mayonnaise and cider vinegar.

Waldorf Salad

Serves 8

6 crunchy apples
⅛ cup fresh lemon juice
3 celery stalks, chopped

½ cup walnuts, chopped
8 lettuce leaves

Cut apples into eight pieces and sprinkle with lemon juice to keep color from turning brown. Combine the apples, celery, and walnuts. Spoon mixture onto lettuce leaves. Top with Orange Yogurt Dressing and toss gently.

Lentil Salad

Serves 4

1 cup lentils
2 cups water
½ teaspoon sea salt
¼ cup celery, finely
  chopped
¼ cup red onion, finely
  chopped

¼ cup black olives, finely
  chopped
2 to 3 tablespoons
  wine vinegar
3 tablespoons olive oil
1 teaspoon basil

Wash lentils and combine with water in a pot. Cook for ½ hour or until lentils are soft. In a bowl, combine cooked lentils with salt, celery, red onion and black olives. Toss with wine vinegar, olive oil, and basil.

Tofu-Wild Rice Salad

Serves 4

6 ounces tofu
2 cups cooked wild rice
3 scallions, chopped

¼ to ½ cup parsley,
  minced
½ green pepper, minced

Cut tofu into bite-sized pieces. Combine with all other ingredients in a bowl. Top with Red Raspberry Vinagrette Dressing. Note: Brown rice may be substituted for wild rice.

Brown Rice and Tofu Salad

Serves 4

2 cups cooked brown rice
8 ounces tofu, diced
1 green onion, diced
¼ cup raisins
1½ ounces almonds,
  blanched

¼ cup peas, cooked
¼ cup green pepper,
  chopped
¼ cup celery, chopped

Combine all ingredients in a bowl. The salad may be dressed with Terry's Rice Vinegar Vinaigrette.

Buckwheat and Pasta Salad

Serves 4

2 cups cooked buckwheat
1 cup cooked pasta (bows or
  fusilli)
¼ cup black olives,
  chopped and pitted

2 green onions, chopped
8 cherry tomatoes
¼ carrot, shredded
¼ head cabbage, shredded

Combine all ingredients in a bowl. Serve with Vinaigrette Dressing.

Salad Dressings

Dressing can make or break a salad. Take the time to make your own; the dressings you create will be fresher, healthier, and tastier. You can be sure you're getting the best ingredients with just the flavors you like.

Low-Stress Ranch Dressing

Makes 2 cups

1 envelope Ranch Dressing
  Mix
1 cup plain soy yogurt
  (nondairy)

½ cup nondairy milk (soy
  or other base)
½ cup mayonnaise

Combine all ingredients and mix well with a whisk or fork. This recipe helps lower the fat content of the dressing significantly while maintaining its delicious flavor.

Louie Dressing

Makes 2½ cups

½ cup mayonnaise
½ cup plain soy yogurt
½ cup ketchup
2 teaspoons honey (or other
  sweetener)

2 teaspoons cider vinegar
2 tablespoons relish
½ teaspoon Dijon mustard

Combine all ingredients in a bowl. Mix until smooth. Serve chilled over shrimp salad or other seafood salad.

Italian Parmesan Dressing

Makes 1½ cups

1 cup olive oil
⅓ cup red wine vinegar
2 tablespoons lemon juice
3 tablespoons parmesan soy
    cheese

½ clove garlic, crushed
1½ teaspoons basil
1½ teaspoons oregano
¼ teaspoon black pepper

Combine all ingredients and blend well.

Vinaigrette Dressing

Makes 1½ cups

1 cup olive oil
½ cup cider vinegar
2 teaspoons Dijon mustard

1 clove garlic, minced
¼ teaspoon black pepper
¼ teaspoon sea salt

Combine all ingredients and blend well.

Red Raspberry Vinaigrette

Makes ½ cup

3 tablespoons raspberry vinegar
4 tablespoons olive oil
1 teaspoon honey (or other sweetener)

Combine all ingredients in a cruet, and mix well.

Balsamic-Honey Dressing

Makes approximately 6 ounces

4 tablespoons Balsamic
  vinegar
4 tablespoons olive oil

3 tablespoons honey
½ teaspoon Dijon mustard

Combine all ingredients and mix well. Serve on spinach salad or other salad requiring a sweeter dressing.

Orange Yogurt Dressing

Makes 1½ cups

1 cup vanilla soy yogurt
½ cup orange juice

Blend well and serve with fruit salads.

Strawberry Yogurt Dressing

Makes 1½ cups

½ cup strawberries
1 teaspoon honey
1 cup plain soy yogurt

Purée strawberries and honey. Combine with yogurt and blend well. Serve with fruit salads.

Miso Salad Dressing

Makes 1½ cups

1 cup warm water
1 teaspoon miso
½ garlic clove, minced
¼ to ½ lemon, juiced

dash cayenne pepper
½ cup tahini
    (sesame butter)

Dissolve miso in warm water. Place in blender with remaining ingredients. Blend until smooth. (For thinner consistency, add more water. For dip consistency, use less water.)

Variations: 1 to 3 teaspoons seasoned rice wine vinegar may be added for sweetness.

Terry's Rice Vinegar Vinaigrette

Makes 1 cup

¼ cup canola oil
¼ cup seasoned rice
    vinegar
¼ cup water
1 to 2 tablespoons lime juice
1 tablespoon plus
    1 teaspoon Dijon mustard

1 tablespoon chives,
    finely chopped
1 tablespoon shallots,
    minced
½ teaspoon tarragon

Combine all ingredients and mix well. Serve on mixed green salads.

Sandwiches

There's a world of fresh vegetables waiting for the creative hand to pack into portable meals. Where would we be without these quick, easy lunches that go anywhere anytime, from the office to picnic grounds to school lunchboxes?

Vegetarian Sandwich Filling *Serves 1*

4 slices avocado
4 slices carrot
2 slices red onion (thin)

2 slices tomato
1 slice soy American or
   Cheddar cheese

Layer in sandwich and serve. Garnish with sprouts, which make a wonderful addition to the sandwich, if desired.

Avocado Sandwich Spread *Serves 2*

1 avocado, mashed
2 tablespoons mayonnaise
½ teaspoon lemon juice

½ teaspoon paprika
2 leaves romaine lettuce
2 slices tomato

Peel and mash avocado in bowl with fork. Add mayonnaise, lemon juice, and paprika, mixing thoroughly. Serve on thin slices of bread or rye crackers with tomato and lettuce.

Sesame Butter and Strawberry Jam

Serves 1

3 tablespoons raw sesame butter
3 tablespoons strawberry jam (no added sugar)

Spread in sandwich and serve.

Tuna Sandwich

Serves 2

6 ounces canned albacore
   tuna in water, drained
2 to 3 teaspoons low-fat
   mayonnaise

2 teaspoons green onions
2 tablespoons celery,
   chopped

Combine all ingredients in a bowl and mix thoroughly.
Serve on bread or crackers.

Almond Butter and Peach Jam

Serves 1

3 tablespoons raw almond butter
3 tablespoons peach jam (no added sugar)

Spread in sandwich and serve.

Note: Other fruit jams such as apricot, strawberry, and
raspberry are also delicious with almond butter.

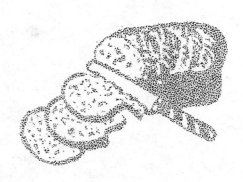

Eggplant Sandwich Spread   *Serves 4*

1 eggplant, medium   2 tablespoons olive oil
1 onion, finely chopped   ¼ cup black olives,
1 cup celery, diced   chopped
1 lemon, juiced   1 garlic clove, minced

Bake eggplant at 350°F until soft. Remove skin and mash to a
smooth texture. Combine all other ingredients and let stand at
least 5 minutes. Combine eggplant with other ingredients; mix
thoroughly. Chill and serve on bread or crackers.

Grains and Starches

Carbohydrates are an important source of energy and the
staple of every nation's diet. Experiment with new grains and
see how easy and satisfying it is to make buckwheat, rice,
potato, and bean dishes.

BASIC RECIPES

Brown Rice   *Serves 4*

1 cup brown rice
2 cups cold water

Wash rice with cold water. Combine with water in a pot. Bring
to a rapid boil. Turn heat to low, cover pot, and cook without
stirring for 25 to 35 minutes, until rice is soft. Resist the
temptation to check before 20 minutes since that lets out too
much steam. Remove cooked rice from burner and let sit for
10 minutes before opening lid. Fluff with fork and serve.

Wild Rice

Serves 2 to 4

⅔ cup wild rice
2½ cups cold water
½ teaspoon sea salt

Wash rice with cold water. Combine all ingredients in a
cooking pot and bring to a rapid boil. Turn to low, cover, and
cook without stirring until rice is tender (about 45 minutes)
but not mushy. Uncover and fluff with a fork. Cook an
additional 5 minutes, then serve.

Kasha

Serves 2 to 4

1 cup kasha (buckwheat groats)
2 cups water
pinch salt

Bring ingredients to a boil, lower heat, and simmer for 25
minutes or until soft. The grain should be fluffy, like rice.

Baked Sweet Potato

Serves 4

4 sweet potatoes
1 tablespoon canola oil
1 tablespoon flax oil for each potato

Preheat oven to 400°F. Wash the potatoes, then rub with canola
oil. Bake for 45 to 60 minutes, or until soft when pierced with a
fork. Garnish with flax oil. Honey, maple syrup, or chopped
raw pecans may also be used as garnishes.

Baked Potato

Serves 4

4 russet or Idaho potatoes
1 tablespoon vegetable oil
1 tablespoon flax oil (each potato)

Preheat oven to 400°F. Wash potatoes, rub with vegetable oil, and bake for 45 to 60 minutes, until soft when pierced with a fork. Garnish with flax oil. Other garnishes include chopped green onions, soy cheese, and low-salt salsa.

Baked Yams

Serves 4

4 yams
1 teaspoon maple syrup (if desired) for each yam

Preheat oven to 400°F. Wash yams and bake for 45 to 60 minutes, until soft when pierced with a fork. Top with maple syrup if desired.

Adzuki Beans

Serves 4

1 cup adzuki beans
4 cups water
½ teaspoon sea salt

Wash beans. Place in pot with water and salt. Bring water to boil, cover, and simmer for 2 hours or until beans are tender.

SIDE DISHES

Kasha with Flax Oil and Tamari

Serves 2

1 cup cooked kasha
3 tablespoons flax oil
1 teaspoon tamari

Combine all ingredients and serve.

Mashed Potatoes

Serves 4

4 large russet potatoes
¾ cup nondairy milk
2 to 3 tablespoons flax oil

1 teaspoon Bragg's Liquid
   Aminos

Peel potatoes and cut into large chunks. Steam for 20 minutes or until soft. Combine potatoes and nondairy milk in a food processor and blend until smooth. Add flax oil and Bragg's; mix well.

Sweet Potato Purée *Serves 4*

3 large sweet potatoes
2 cups nondairy milk
6 ounces raw pecans,
    chopped
1 cup pineapple, in chunks

3 tablespoons maple syrup
2 tablespoons flax oil
¼ teaspoon cinnamon
½ teaspoon guar gum

Remove skin from sweet potatoes and cut into large chunks.
Steam for 15 minutes or until potatoes are soft. Place sweet
potatoes in a food processor and whip into a purée, slowly
adding the nondairy milk. Remove from food processor and
place in a large bowl. Mix pecans, pineapple, maple syrup, flax
oil, and cinnamon into the sweet potatoes and blend well. Add
guar gum and blend. Serve.

Mashed Potatos and Turnips *Serves 4*

2 cups white potatoes, sliced
1 cup turnips, sliced

½ cup nondairy milk
2 tablespoons flax oil

Steam potatoes for 15 minutes, add turnips, and continue to
steam for 30 minutes or until vegetables are soft. Remove from
heat and place in mixing bowl. Add nondairy milk and beat
with electric mixer until smooth. Add flax oil and blend well
into potato-turnip mixture with large spoon.

Low-Fat Sweet Potato Fries

Serves 4

2 large sweet potatoes
2 tablespoons canola oil

Peel sweet potatoes and slice lengthwise into thin, julienne string potatoes. Pour canola oil into a wok or deep frying pan over high heat. Immediately add sweet potato strips and cook for 4 minutes or until sweet potatoes soften brown.

Spicy Near Beer Beans

Serves 4

2 cups pinto beans
26 ounces (3¼ cups) Near Beer
1 cup vegetable broth
1 onion, chopped
2 cloves garlic, minced
1 teaspoon chili powder
1 teaspoon allspice
½ teaspoon cinnamon
½ teaspoon oregano
½ teaspoon cumin
1 tablespoon maple syrup

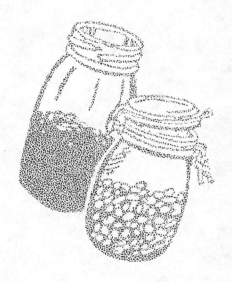

Rinse beans and place in cooking pot. Add 20 ounces of Near Beer; then add the vegetable broth, onion, garlic, chili powder, allspice, cinnamon, oregano, cumin, and maple syrup. Bring to a boil and cook for 3 to 3½ hours or until beans are soft. Add 6 more ounces of Near Beer during the cooking process so beans stay moist. Alternatively, you can cook the beans and spices overnight in a crock pot.

Rice and Mushrooms

Serves 4

2¼ cups vegetable broth
2 tablespoons Madeira wine
1 cup brown rice blend
⅛ teaspoon saffron
1 medium shallot, minced

4 medium white
  mushrooms, chopped
¾ cup wild mushrooms,
  coarsely chopped
1 to 1¼ teaspoons canola oil

Bring vegetable broth and 2 tablespoons of Madeira to a boil; add brown rice blend and saffron. Reduce heat to low, cover pot, and cook for 45 minutes or until rice is fluffy. Sauté shallots, white mushrooms, and wild mushrooms in canola oil for 3 to 4 minutes. Combine with rice and serve.

Risotto Milanese

Serves 4 to 6

1 cup white rice
2 cups vegetable broth
1 tablespoon canola oil
¾ cup green peas
1 shallot, minced

10 small mushrooms, diced
⅛ teaspoon sea salt
3 tablespoons white wine
2 tablespoons soy parmesan
  cheese

Combine rice and vegetable broth in a cooking pot. Bring to a boil. Cover pot, and turn heat to low, and cook for 20 minutes or until rice is fluffy. Sauté green peas, shallot, and mushrooms in canola oil until vegetables are soft. Add sea salt and mix. Transfer to a serving dish, add white wine, and sprinkle with soy parmesan cheese. Mix well and serve.

Vegetables

The rule of thumb for vegetables: eat as many as you can, as often as you like, as fresh as possible. Do try to have greens often but don't overlook the cornucopia of other treasures in this abundant Earth garden.

Vegetable Purée #1
Serves 4

3 to 4 carrots, chopped
⅛ head cabbage, chopped
1 cup peas

Steam carrots for 15 minutes, add other vegetables and steam for 15 more minutes until soft. Place in blender and purée. Slowly add water until smooth and creamy.

Vegetables Purée #2
Serves 4

1 medium beet, chopped
4 summer squash, chopped

Steam beet for 15 minutes. Add squash to the pot and steam the vegetables together for 15 more minutes until soft. Purée in blender.

Steamed Kale

Serves 4

1 bunch kale
  (stems removed), chopped
1 lemon, juiced

2 to 3 tablespoons olive oil
pinch of sea salt

Steam kale until tender. Dress with lemon juice, olive oil, and sea salt. Kale is an excellent vegetable for women since it is a good source of calcium. I recommend eating it frequently. Swiss chard and mustard greens, two other excellent vegetables for women, can be prepared and dressed the same way.

Steamed Cabbage

Serves 4

1 small head cabbage, quartered
1 teaspoon olive oil
1 teaspoon parsley, chopped

Steam cabbage until tender. Sprinkle with olive oil and parsley.

Broccoli with Lemon

Serves 4

1 pound broccoli
½ lemon, juiced
4 tablespoons flax oil

Cut broccoli into small flowerettes. Steam for 6 minutes or until tender. Squeeze lemon juice over broccoli and add the flax oil. Mix and serve. For a different taste, try substituting Bragg's Liquid Aminos for the lemon juice.

Cauliflower with Flax Oil

Serves 4

1 medium head cauliflower
4 tablespoons flax oil
1 teaspoon salt substitute

Break the cauliflower into small flowerettes. Steam 10 minutes or until tender. Toss with flax oil and salt substitute for a buttery taste.

Savory Bean Sprouts

Serves 4

1 cup chicken stock
1½ cup bean sprouts
1 cup mushrooms, sliced

Heat chicken stock over low heat for 5 minutes. Add bean sprouts and mushrooms. Simmer for 10 minutes.

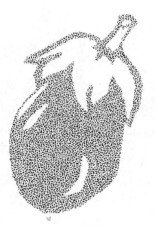

Zucchini and Eggplant

Serves 4

2 medium zucchini, sliced
1 cup eggplant, cubed
1 small onion, chopped
1 clove garlic, minced

½ teaspoon basil
½ teaspoon oregano
1 tablespoon olive oil
⅛ teaspoon salt

Sauté zucchini, eggplant, and onion in a frying pan with a small amount of water. Add remaining ingredients. Cook until tender, stirring constantly.

Zucchini with Scallions

Serves 4

2 teaspoons safflower oil
2 medium zucchini, diced
2 teaspoons scallions,
    chopped

½ clove garlic, minced
1 teaspoon dried basil
1 teaspoon oregano

Heat oil in frying pan on medium heat. Add all ingredients to pan. Cook until tender, stirring constantly.

Steamed Leeks

Serves 4

8 medium leeks
2 tablespoons red onion, minced

Remove and discard green tops and rinse leeks thoroughly. Cut each root end into two pieces. Steam 15 to 20 minutes until tender. Sprinkle onion on top before serving.

Celery Julienne

Serves 4

6 stalks celery
2 tablespoons sweet red pepper, chopped

Cut the celery into small strips (like French-fried potatoes). Steam for 15 to 20 minutes, until tender. Drain and toss with red pepper.

Green Beans with Almonds

Serves 4

1 pound green beans
2 ounces raw almonds,
  chopped

2 tablespoons flax oil
¼ teaspoon salt substitute

Steam green beans until tender. Toss with the almond bits, flax
oil, and sea salt for a buttery flavor. If you don't care for the
taste of flax oil, substitute a vinaigrette dressing.

Green Peas and Onions

Serves 4

1 cup water
1 cup green peas
½ cup onions, diced

Boil water, then turn heat to low. Add peas and onion and
simmer for 20 minutes or until peas are tender. Drain any
excess water.

Summer Squash and Peas

Serves 4

1 cup peas
2 to 3 small summer squash, diced

Steam peas for 10 minutes. Add squash and steam vegetables
together for 15 minutes or until tender. Drain and serve.

Diced Carrots with Peas

Serves 4

1½ cups chicken stock
1 cup green peas
1 cup carrots, diced

Heat chicken stock to a boil, then turn heat to low. Add peas and carrots and simmer for 30 minutes or until vegetables are tender.

Whipped Acorn Squash

Serves 4

2 acorn squash
¼ to ⅓ cup apple juice
pinch cinnamon, ground

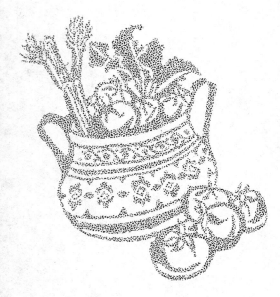

Peel and cut acorn squash into large pieces. Steam until tender. Place in food processor, add apple juice and cinnamon, and purée. You may also want to add water in small amounts until texture is smooth and creamy.

Maple Sugar Carrots

Serves 4

12 small carrots, cleaned and sliced
4 tablespoons pecans, chopped
1 tablespoon maple syrup

Steam carrots until soft. Combine with pecans and drizzle with maple syrup.

Creamed Spinach

Serves 4

1¾ cups steamed spinach
2 tablespoons canola oil
¼ cup yellow onion, finely chopped
1 tablespoon unbleached flour or rice flour

1 cup nondairy milk
2 tablespoons apple juice
⅛ teaspoon paprika
¼ teaspoon nutmeg
¼ teaspoon sea salt
¼ teaspoon guar gum

Blend steamed spinach in a food processor until finely puréed. Heat canola oil over medium heat and add onions. Cook onions until lightly golden brown. Add flour to frying pan and blend well with oil and onion mixture. Add nondairy milk, apple juice, paprika, nutmeg, sea salt, and guar gum. Add spinach and blend thoroughly.

Butternut Squash Puree

Serves 4

2 butternut squash, 2 pounds each
1 carrot, sliced
2 ounces yellow onion, finely chopped

2 tablespoons canola oil
2½ cups nondairy milk
¼ teaspoon ginger
¾ teaspoon mace
2 tablespoons maple syrup

Peel butternut squash with a potato peeler and cut into 1-inch squares (be sure to discard the seeds). Place the squash and carrot in a steamer and cook for 20 to 25 minutes or until vegetables are soft. As the vegetables steam, heat canola oil in a frying pan over medium heat; add onions and sauté for 3 to 5 minutes or until onion softens. Place squash, carrots, onion, and nondairy milk in a food processor and blend well. Then add ginger, mace, and maple syrup and mix until flavors are well blended.

Vegetarian Main Courses

Explore exotic new dishes and experience a world of flavors right in your own kitchen. You can experience the delights of Italian Pesto, Russian Stroganoff, Middle Eastern Tabouli, French Orange Sauce, Chinese Stir-Fry, and Mexican Tacos without ever leaving home.

Pasta with Flax Oil and Garlic   *Serves 4*

1 pound nonwheat pasta
  (rice, corn, or buckwheat)
1 clove garlic, minced
4 tablespoons flax oil

1 teaspoon basil
½ teaspoon sea salt
1 tablespoon soy parmesan
  cheese

Cook pasta until tender. Top with garlic, flax oil, basil, salt, and soy parmesan. Mix well and serve.

Pesto Rice and Tofu   *Serves 4*

4 cups cooked brown rice
1 cup firm tofu, diced
pesto, to taste

Combine rice and tofu in a large bowl. Top with the desired amount of pesto (see following recipe). Mix and serve.

Pesto Sauce

Serves 4

2 large cloves garlic, minced
3 cups fresh basil leaves, chopped
½ cup almonds, chopped

2 tablespoons parmesan cheese, grated
pinch of sea salt
½ cup olive oil

Combine garlic, basil, almonds, cheese, and salt in a food processor until well mixed. Slowly add olive oil until mixture forms a smooth paste. Pesto may be refrigerated for a few weeks and also freezes well. It is excellent as a sauce for rice or pasta.

Linguini with Red Clam Sauce

Serves 4

½ cup olive oil
5 cloves garlic
2 large cloves shallots
4 cups tomatoes, coarsely chopped
1 sprig parsley, chopped

½ teaspoon dry basil
½ teaspoon dry oregano
½ teaspoon sea salt
2 cans (5-ounce) clams
½ pound dry linguini

Place olive oil, garlic, and shallots in frying pan. Cook over medium heat for 5 minutes or until golden brown. Add the tomatoes and clam juice from the cans. Turn heat to low and simmer; add parsley, basil, oregano, sea salt, and clams; cook for 20 minutes. Bring water to boil in a large pot. Add linguini. Cook for 10 minutes or until al dente. Drain water from linguini and top with clam sauce.

Tofu Stroganoff

1½ cups broccoli
  flowerettes
2 tablespoons canola oil
1 pound mushrooms, sliced
4 tablespoons shallots,
  minced
2 cloves garlic, minced
1 cup firm tofu, sliced
  in 1-inch strips
2 cups soy sour cream

⅓ cup Madeira wine
½ teaspoon paprika
2 to 2½ teaspoons tamari
  soy sauce
⅛ teaspoon black pepper
¼ teaspoon Worcestershire
  sauce
4½ cups wide egg
  noodles, cooked and well
  drained

Steam broccoli flowerettes for 6 minutes or until slightly tender. Sauté mushrooms, shallots, and garlic in canola oil until slightly golden brown. Add tofu and broccoli and continue to sauté for 2 more minutes. Add soy sour cream and Madeira wine and mix well. Finally, add paprika, tamari, black pepper, and Worcestershire sauce to the mixture and blend well. Serve over warm egg noodles.

Pasta with Chickpeas

Serves 4

2 cups cooked nonwheat
    pasta (corn, quinoa, or rice)
1 cup cooked chickpeas
    (garbanzo beans)
⅔ cup steamed broccoli,
    chopped
¼ cup red onion, diced

¼ cup green pepper, diced
½ teaspoon basil
½ teaspoon tarragon
3 tablespoons olive oil
½ lemon, juiced
⅛ teaspoon salt

Combine all ingredients in a large bowl. Mix well, chill, and serve.

Two-Bean Dish

Serves 2

¾ cup cooked black beans
¾ cup cooked lentils or
    Great Northern beans
¼ red pepper, diced
¼ small red onion, diced

¼ cup celery, diced
6 leaves romaine lettuce
1 cup cooked brown rice
2 tablespoons green onions,
    chopped

In two separate bowls, combine each bean portion with one half of the red pepper, red onion, and celery. Mix well. Arrange leaves of romaine lettuce on a serving dish. Place brown rice in the center and arrange beans on either side. Sprinkle with chopped green onions and dress with oil and vinegar or your favorite vinaigrette dressing.

Tofu Sausage and Mushroom Pizza

Serves 2 to 4

1 pizza crust, (12-inch)
1½ teaspoons olive oil
¾ cup low-salt
  tomato sauce
1 large tomato
2 tofu sausages*, thinly
  sliced

8 mushrooms, sliced
1 small red onion, sliced
½ teaspoon dry basil
½ teaspoon dry oregano
¼ teaspoon marjoram
½ cup soy mozzarella
  cheese, grated (optional)

Preheat oven to 450°F. Drizzle oil on pizza crust. Spread tomato sauce evenly over the crust. Cut tomato into thin wedges and distribute evenly over crust. Distribute tofu sausage, mushroom, and onion slices over crust. Sprinkle with basil, oregano, and marjoram. Bake in oven for 16 minutes or until crust is golden brown. Add soy mozzarella and continue to bake for 4 more minutes.

*Note: Tofu sausage is available in many supermarkets under the Morningstar Farms label.

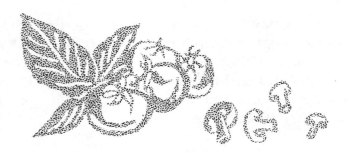

Two-Pepper Pizza   *Serves 2 to 4*

1 pizza crust, (12-inch)
1½ teaspoons olive oil
¾ cup low-salt
  tomato sauce
1 green pepper, chopped
1 red pepper, chopped

1 small red onion, chopped
8 mushrooms, sliced
½ teaspoon dry basil
½ teaspoon dry oregano
4 tablespoons soy parmesan
  cheese

Preheat oven to 450°F. Drizzle oil over pizza crust, then spread
tomato sauce evenly over crust. Distribute green and red
peppers evenly over crust. Add onions and mushrooms.
Sprinkle with oregano and basil. Bake in oven for 20 minutes.
Top with soy parmesan and bake for an additional 2 minutes.

Artichoke and Olive Pizza   *Serves 2 to 4*

1 pizza crust, (12-inch)
1½ teaspoons olive oil
¾ cup low-salt
  tomato sauce
1 large tomato
6 cooked artichoke hearts,
  chopped

10 black olives, chopped
½ small red onion, sliced
½ green pepper, chopped
½ teaspoon dry basil
½ teaspoon dry oregano
½ cup mozzarella cheese,
  grated (optional)

Preheat oven to 450°F. Drizzle oil on pizza crust. Spread
tomato sauce evenly over crust. Cut tomato into thin wedges
and distribute evenly over crust. Distribute artichoke hearts,
olives, onion, and green pepper over crust. Sprinkle with basil
and oregano. Bake in oven for 16 minutes or until crust is
golden brown. Add soy mozzarella cheese and continue to
bake for 4 more minutes.

Stuffed Peppers   *Serves 6*

6 green peppers   ½ cup low-sodium
¾ cup celery, diced   tomato juice
1 cup onions, chopped   ¼ teaspoon sea salt
2½ cups cooked   2 cups tomato sauce (amount
   brown rice   may be adjusted to taste)

Preheat oven to 350°F. Scoop out peppers. Mix all other
ingredients except tomato sauce. Fill peppers with mixture.
Place peppers in baking dish. Pour tomato sauce over peppers
and bake uncovered for 45 minutes. Serve hot. (See recipe
below for tomato sauce).

Tomato Sauce   *Serves 2 to 4*

2 tablespoons canola oil   1 can (6 ounces) tomato
1 clove garlic, minced   paste
½ small onion, chopped   1 teaspoon basil
½ green pepper, diced   1 teaspoon oregano
2 cups tomatoes, chopped   ½ teaspoon sea salt

Sauté garlic, onion, and green pepper together in oil over
medium heat until tender. Add remaining ingredients and
cook on low for 15 minutes.

Kasha with Zucchini   *Serve 2 to 4*

3 cups cooked kasha
1½ cups zucchini, sliced
½ cup onions, chopped

¼ cup olive oil
1½ cups tomato sauce

Sauté zucchini and onions in olive oil until tender. Combine with kasha. Cook on low heat for 10 minutes. Mix well with tomato sauce (see preceding recipe) and serve.

Kasha and Kidney Beans   *Serves 2*

2 cups cooked kasha
¾ cup cooked kidney
   beans
1 zucchini, sliced
⅓ onion, chopped

3 tablespoons olive oil
¾ cup low-salt tomato
   sauce (see Stuffed Pepper
   recipe for sauce)

Combine kasha and kidney beans and set aside. Sauté zucchini and onion in olive oil until slightly brown. Combine with kasha and kidney beans. Top with tomato sauce and serve.

Rice and Almond Tabouli

Serves 6

2 cups cooked brown rice
1 cup parsley, chopped
½ cup fresh mint, chopped
½ medium red onion,
  diced
1 medium tomato, diced

1 heaping tablespoon
  almonds, chopped
1 lemon, juiced
2 tablespoons olive oil
1 teaspoon cumin
1 teaspoon oregano
¼ teaspoon salt

Place rice in a bowl. Mix in parsley, mint, red onion, tomato, and chopped almonds. Combine these ingredients well. Add lemon juice and olive oil and mix. Add cumin, oregano, and salt to the salad and mix well. This is the ultimate delicious and healthy tabouli recipe. It is great served with hummus and tahini and a few Greek black olives.

Hummus and Tahini

Serves 4

¾ cup raw sesame seeds,
  unhulled
1 cup water or cooking
  liquid from beans
1¾ cup cooked garbanzo
  beans

1 clove garlic
1 lemon, juiced
1 to 2 tablespoons olive oil
  (to taste)
¼ teaspoon salt

To make tahini, grind sesame seeds into a powder using a seed or coffee grinder. Place to one side in a dish. Raw sesame butter may be substituted, which is available from most health food stores. Combine water, garbanzo beans, ground sesame seeds, garlic, lemon juice, olive oil, and salt in a food processor. Blend until smooth. Serve as a dip with pita bread, rye bread, and fresh vegetables.

Acorn Squash with Wild Rice Stuffing   *Serves 4*

2 acorn squash, halved

Preheat oven to 375°F. Place acorn squash, cut side down, in ½ cup of water in a Pyrex baking or other cooking dish. Bake for 35 minutes or until soft. Fill with rice stuffing (see recipe below) and serve.

Wild Rice Stuffing

3 tablespoons canola oil
1 small red onion, chopped
1 clove garlic, minced
⅓ cup raisins

1 heaping tablespoon
   pine nuts
pinch sea salt
¼ teaspoon allspice
2 cups cooked wild rice

Precook rice per package instructions. Sauté onions and garlic in canola oil until golden brown. Add raisins and pine nuts. Continue to sauté for 3 to 4 minutes. Combine with cooked wild rice. Add sea salt and allspice to rice mixture and mix well. Add stuffing to individual acorn squash halves just before serving.

Sweet and Sour Cabbage Rolls

Serves 4

3 tablespoons canola oil
1½ cups red onion, chopped
2 cloves garlic, minced
½ cup mushrooms, chopped
3¼ cups cooked wild rice

½ cup raisins
½ cup firm tofu, finely diced
½ teaspoon paprika
¼ teaspoon sea salt
1 medium head green cabbage

Preheat oven to 375°F. Heat canola oil in a frying pan over medium heat. Add onion and garlic and cook until slightly brown. Add mushrooms and cook for 2 minutes. Add wild rice, raisins, tofu, paprika, and sea salt. Cook for 3 to 5 minutes. Place to one side. Remove core of cabbage. Place cabbage on a steamer in a large pot and steam for 9 minutes or until leaves are tender. Remove from heat. Gently remove 8 leaves from cabbage and lay on flat surface. Spoon 4 tablespoons of filling onto each leaf. Roll leaf up into egg roll shape, tucking in ends of cabbage. Place each cabbage roll in a baking dish. Cover amply with 4 to 5 cups Sweet and Sour Sauce (see following recipe). Bake for 30 to 35 minutes and serve.

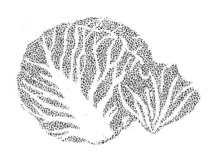

Sweet and Sour Sauce

Serves 4

3 tablespoons canola oil
¾ cup red onion, chopped
1 can (28-ounce) whole
    tomatoes, cut into large
    chunks

½ cup tomato paste
½ cup apple juice
½ teaspoon cinnamon

Heat canola oil in a pan over medium heat. Add onion and cook until golden brown. Add tomatoes, tomato paste, apple juice, and cinnamon; cook over low heat for 5 minutes. Use as sauce for cabbage rolls.

Wild Rice and Spinach with Hazelnut Sauce

Serves 6

2 tablespoons canola oil
1 cup red onion, chopped
2 cloves garlic, minced
½ cup mushrooms,
    chopped
4 cups cooked wild rice

½ cup firm tofu, finely
    diced
¼ teaspoon sea salt
¼ teaspoon paprika
2 bunches spinach, washed
    and stems removed

Heat canola oil in a frying pan over medium heat. Add onion, garlic, and mushrooms; sauté for 3 to 5 minutes or until vegetables are slightly golden brown. Add wild rice, tofu, sea salt, and paprika and cook over low heat for 5 minutes. Blend the mixture well and set aside.

Place spinach in a steamer and steam for 12 minutes. Divide spinach into 6 portions and place on serving dish. Mound wild rice and tofu mixture on top of each bed of spinach, then top with Hazelnut Sauce (see following recipe).

Hazelnut Sauce

Makes 2½ cups

1 cup raw hazelnuts, shelled
1 tablespoon canola oil
1 small onion, diced

1 clove garlic, minced
¾ cup tawny port wine
¾ cup spring water

Place hazelnuts in a food processor and grind to a fine consistency. Heat canola oil in a frying pan over medium heat and add onion and garlic. Cook until golden brown. Add tawny port, water, and hazelnuts to the pan and continue to cook over medium heat for 5 to 7 minutes. Be sure to stir continuously so mixture is well blended and alcohol cooks off. Transfer sauce to food processor and blend again. Serve over bed of wild rice, tofu, and spinach.

Wild Rice and Tofu with Orange-Currant Sauce

Serves 4

3 tablespoons canola oil
1 cup red onion, chopped
2 cloves garlic, minced
½ cup mushrooms, sliced
3 cups cooked wild rice

½ cup currants
½ cup firm tofu, diced
¼ teaspoon sea salt
⅛ teaspoon black pepper

Heat canola oil over medium heat in a frying pan. Add onion and garlic and cook until slightly brown. Add mushrooms and cook for 2 minutes. Add wild rice, currants, tofu, salt, and pepper and cook for 3 to 5 minutes. Transfer to a large serving dish and top with Orange-Currant Sauce (see following recipe). Garnish plates with orange slices for an attractive presentation.

Orange-Currant Sauce

Makes 2 cups

1 cup intensely flavored
  vegetable broth
1 teaspoon cornstarch or
  arrowroot powder
1 tablespoon red currant jelly
1 cup orange juice
¼ teaspoon orange zest
  (grated orange rind)

1 teaspoon sweetener
  (artificial sweetener may
  be used)
½ teaspoon guar gum
1 to 2 tablespoons orange-
  flavored liqueur

Place vegetable broth and cornstarch in a cooking pot and mix
together. Add red currant jelly and blend into broth. Add
orange juice, orange zest, and sweetener and cook over
medium heat for another 3 to 4 minutes. Add guar gum and
continue to cook over medium-low heat for 3 to 4 minutes,
stirring occasionally until sauce thickens. Mix in orange-
flavored liqueur. Serve over wild rice-tofu dish.

Wild Rice and Tofu with Raspberry Sauce

Serves 4

3 tablespoons canola oil
1 cup red onion, chopped
2 cloves garlic, minced
½ cup mushrooms, sliced

3 cups cooked wild rice
½ cup firm tofu, diced
¼ teaspoon sea salt

Heat canola oil in a frying pan over medium heat. Add onion
and garlic and cook until slightly brown. Add mushrooms and
cook for 2 minutes. Add wild rice, tofu, and sea salt and cook
for 3 to 5 minutes. Transfer to a large serving dish and top with
Raspberry Sauce (see following recipe).

Raspberry Sauce

Makes 1½ cups

1½ cups frozen
  raspberries
1 cup orange juice
1 tablespoon honey

2 teaspoons artificial
  sweetener
½ teaspoon guar gum

Purée raspberries, orange juice, honey, and artificial sweetener in a food processor. Transfer to a sauce pot and cook over medium heat. Add guar gum, sprinkling it over the sauce. Stir the sauce frequently as it thickens. Cook for several minutes. Serve over wild rice-tofu dish.

Mixed Vegetable Stir-Fry

Serves 4

¼ cup olive oil
2 cups zucchini
2 medium onions, sliced
1 cup bean sprouts

⅓ cup celery, thinly sliced
¼ cup green onions
2 cups cooked brown rice

Place olive oil in pan over medium heat. Add zucchini, onions, sprouts, celery, and green onions. Cover and sauté until vegetables are slightly tender. Do not overcook. Serve over brown rice.

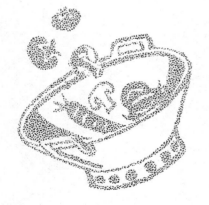

Stir-Fry with Snow Peas

Serves 4

⅓ cup celery, diced
⅓ cup red pepper, diced
1 cup snow peas, steamed
¼ cup water
1 teaspoon sesame or
  safflower oil

¾ cup tofu, diced
3 cups cooked brown rice
tamari, to taste

Combine celery, red pepper, and snow peas in a large frying pan with water and oil. Cook over low flame for 5 minutes adding tofu for the last 3 minutes of cooking. (Add extra water to pan if needed.) Add rice to pan and mix. Heat for 5 minutes or until warm. Transfer to serving dish and toss with tamari.

Tofu and Almond Stir-Fry

Serves 4

¾ cups firm tofu, cubed
1 cup raw almonds,
  chopped
¼ yellow onion
½ red pepper, chopped

¼ cup water
1 teaspoon sesame or
  safflower oil
3 cups cooked brown rice
1 teaspoon tamari

Combine tofu, almonds, onion, and red peppers in a large frying pan with water and oil. Cook over low flame for 5 minutes. (Add extra water to pan if needed.) Add rice to pan and mix. Heat for 5 minutes or until warm. Transfer to serving dish and toss with tamari.

Tofu and Millet Stir-Fry   *Serves 4*

¾ cup tofu, cubed
¼ yellow onion, sliced
1 cup green beans, steamed
¼ cup water

1 teaspoon sesame or
   safflower oil
3 cups cooked millet
low-salt soy sauce, to taste

Combine tofu, onion, and green beans in a large frying pan with water and oil. Cook over low heat for 5 minutes. (Add extra water to pan if needed.) Add millet and mix. Heat for 5 minutes or until warm. Transfer to serving dish and toss with soy sauce.

Tofu and Walnut Rice with Hoisin Sauce   *Serves 4*

½ cup firm tofu, diced
2 tablespoons dry sherry
1 tablespoon low-sodium
   soy sauce
1 tablespoon cornstarch
2 tablespoons canola oil
1 zucchini, sliced

2 green onions, chopped
½ red pepper, sliced
½ cup raw walnuts
2 tablespoons hoisin sauce
2½ cups cooked brown
   rice

Marinate tofu in dry sherry, soy sauce, and cornstarch. Add canola oil to a wok or skillet and heat. Quickly stir-fry the zucchini, green onions, and red pepper. When vegetables are almost cooked, add walnuts, tofu, and hoisin sauce and stir-fry for an additional minute or two until well blended. Combine with rice and serve.

Shrimp and Millet Stir-Fry

Serves 4

¾ cup celery, finely
   chopped
½ cup water
1 teaspoon sesame or
   safflower oil

½ pound shrimp, cooked
   and peeled
3 cups cooked millet
low-salt soy sauce, to taste

Sauté celery in water and oil over low heat for 20 minutes or until tender. Add shrimp and cook for 2 minutes. Transfer to a serving dish and toss with millet and soy sauce.

Salad Tacos

Serves 4

4 corn tortillas
2 cups vegetarian refried
   beans
½ head lettuce
½ small red onion
½ red pepper

1 tomato, sliced
16 black olives, sliced
4 slices soy cheddar cheese,
   sliced in strips
6 ounces Mexican dressing

Spread beans evenly over tortillas. Shred lettuce, onion, and red pepper in food processor; spread over beans. Arrange tomato, olives, and soy cheddar cheese over vegetable mixture and top with Mexican dressing (see following recipe).

Mexican Dressing

Makes 1 cup

1 cup Ranch dressing (see Salad Dressings)
¼ teaspoon cumin
1½ teaspoons chili powder

Combine all ingredients and blend until well mixed.

Vegetarian Tacos

Serves 4

4 corn tortillas
¾ pound cooked pinto
   beans, puréed
½ avocado, thinly sliced
¼ sweet red pepper, diced
1 tomato, diced

¼ red onion, finely
   chopped
½ head red or romaine
   lettuce, chopped
6 tablespoons salsa

Warm tortillas and beans in separate pans. Place tortillas on individual serving dishes and spread with beans. Garnish with avocado, pepper, tomato, and onion, then cover each taco with lettuce and 1½ tablespoons of salsa.

Pasta Primavera

Serves 6

1 carrot, thinly sliced
1 cup broccoli flowerettes
1 red pepper, diced
2 zucchini, thinly sliced
1 cup cauliflower flowerettes
2 to 3 tablespoons olive oil
12 mushrooms, sliced
1 red onion, diced

2 cloves garlic, minced
½ teaspoon sea salt
5 medium tomatoes, sliced
5 tablespoons white wine
2 teaspoons parsley, minced
1 pound cooked spaghetti or
   other pasta

Steam carrot slices for 10 minutes; then add broccoli, red pepper, zucchini, and cauliflower to steamer and continue to cook for 5 minutes or until vegetables are al dente. In a frying pan or wok, sauté olive oil, mushrooms, onions, garlic, and sea salt on high heat for 4 minutes. Add tomatoes, white wine, and parsley and cook for 10 minutes. Add steamed vegetables to the other ingredients, mix well and immediately serve over pasta.

Tomato Eggplant Pasta

Serves 4-6

1 small eggplant, diced
3 tablespoons olive oil
15 medium mushrooms, sliced
3 shallots, minced
2 cloves garlic, minced
5 cups tomatoes, chopped

2 teaspoons basil
½ teaspoon rosemary
2 teaspoons oregano
½ teaspoon sea salt
1 pound cooked linguine or other pasta

Steam eggplant for 3 to 4 minutes; remove from heat and set aside. Sauté mushrooms, shallots, and garlic in olive oil in a frying pan over high heat until the vegetables begin to soften and brown slightly. Add the tomatoes, eggplant, basil, rosemary, oregano, and sea salt and cook over high heat for 5 minutes. Reduce temperature to low and cook for an additional 25 minutes. Serve tomato eggplant sauce over linguine or your favorite pasta.

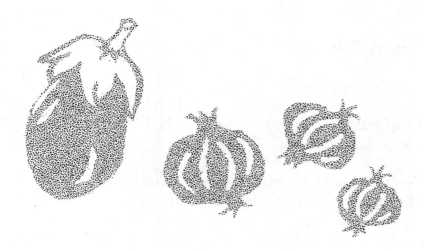

Fish Entrées

With all the essential fatty acids and protein packed in fish, no wonder it's called "brain food." Take care not to serve your fish undercooked or overcooked; just tender enough to melt in your mouth. Saute in a variety of sauces and spices to enhance the flavor. Garnish with fresh parsley.

Poached Salmon #1   *Serves 4*

4 fillets of salmon, 3 ounces each
1 cup water
1 lemon, juiced

Combine water and lemon juice in skillet and heat. Place the salmon in the hot liquid. Cover and poach for 6 to 8 minutes or until the salmon flakes easily with a fork. Remove the fish and keep it warm until you are ready to serve.

Poached Salmon #2   *Serves 4*

4 fillets of salmon, 3 ounces each	¼ cup V-8 juice
1 cup water	1 tablespoon onion, diced
1 lemon, juiced	1 tablespoon carrot, diced

Combine water, lemon juice, and V-8 juice in skillet and heat. Place the salmon in the hot liquid and sprinkle with diced vegetables. Cover and poach for 6 to 8 minutes or until the salmon flakes easily with a fork. Remove the fish and keep it warm until you are ready to serve.

Salmon with Port Wine Sauce

Serves 4

2 small shallots, minced
5 medium mushrooms, diced
1 tablespoon canola oil
6 ounces tawny port
¼ teaspoon guar gum

¼ teaspoon tarragon
1/16 teaspoon sea salt
4 4-ounce salmon fillets,
   grilled

Sauté shallots and mushrooms in canola oil at high heat for 2 minutes or until vegetables are soft. Turn down heat to simmer. Add tawny port, stirring a few times. Immediately add guar gum, tarragon, and sea salt to sauce. Mix and serve over grilled salmon.

Salmon with Kiwi Lime Sauce

Serves 6

4 kiwis, peeled
juice from one lime
6 tablespoons honey
6 4-ounce salmon fillets, grilled

Place kiwis in a blender or food processor with lime juice and honey. Blend until smooth. Serve with grilled salmon.

Broiled Tuna

Serves 4

4 fillets of tuna, 4 ounces each
1 tablespoon canola oil
2 tablespoons lemon juice

Baste the tuna fillets with oil and then sprinkle with lemon juice. Place the tuna in a broiler pan. Broil for 5 to 6 minutes until fish is done to your liking.

Broiled Trout with Dill

Serves 4

2 fresh trout, 8 ounces each
2 tablespoons lemon juice
fresh dill, chopped (dried if fresh is unavailable)

Slice each trout in half and bone. This will make four fillets. Sprinkle the fillets with lemon juice and dill. Place the trout in a broiler pan. Broil for 5 to 6 minutes or until done.

Swordfish with Mustard Sauce

Serves 2

1 shallot, minced
1 tablespoon canola oil
3 tablespoons Dijon (grainy style) mustard
4 ounces nondairy milk
¼ to ½ teaspoon guar gum
2 4-ounce swordfish steaks
2 teaspoons canola oil

Sauté shallot in canola oil for 1 minute on high heat. Add remaining ingredients except guar gum and cook for 1 minute. Add guar gum and stir well.

Sauté swordfish steaks on medium high heat in canola oil for 5 minutes on each side. Cover swordfish with sauce and serve.

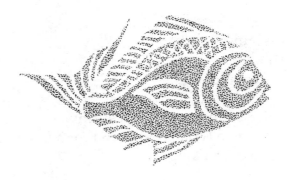

Swordfish with Tomato Caper Sauce   *Serves 2*

1 shallot, minced
2 tomatoes, chopped
2 tablespoons canola oil
2 teaspoons capers

⅛ teaspoon sea salt
2 4-ounce swordfish steaks
2 teaspoons canola oil

Sauté shallots and tomatoes in canola oil at high heat for 3 minutes or until vegetables soften. Then add capers and sea salt and cook for 1 minute more.

Sauté swordfish steaks on medium high heat in canola oil for 5 minutes on each side. Cover swordfish with sauce and serve.

Halibut in Cashew Milk   *Serves 4*

¾ cup fish stock or water
2 tablespoons dry white
  wine
1 shallot, minced
4 halibut steaks, (3 ounces
  each)

½ teaspoon arrowroot
  powder
⅓ cup cashew milk
1 teaspoon lemon juice

Combine fish stock, wine, and shallot in a pot. Heat to boiling. Cover pot and simmer 5 to 10 minutes. Place the halibut in the liquid and poach for 10 minutes. Lift the fish out carefully with a slotted spoon and keep warm. Combine the arrowroot powder with the cashew milk. Mix it slowly into the hot fish stock, stirring constantly until the sauce is the consistency of a thin gravy. Season with lemon juice. Return the halibut to the sauce and simmer for 2 minutes.

Poached Flounder *Serves 4*

2 cups water
2 shallots, chopped
2 sprigs parsley
1 small stalk celery, chopped

1 bay leaf
1 clove
4 flounder fillets, (3 ounces each)

Combine water, shallots, parsley, celery, bay leaf, and clove in a pot. Cover and simmer for 10 minutes. Strain. Gently add the flounder to the liquid. Cover the pot and simmer for 10 minutes or until fish is tender.

Shrimp Marinara *Serves 4*

½ cup olive oil
5 cloves garlic
2 large cloves shallots
4 cups tomatoes, coarsely chopped
1 sprig parsley, chopped
½ teaspoon dry basil

½ teaspoon dry oregano
½ teaspoon sea salt
1 pound cooked and deveined shrimp
1 tablespoon soy parmesan (optional)

Place olive oil, garlic, and shallots in a frying pan and cook over medium heat 5 minutes or until golden brown. Add tomatoes, lower heat and simmer. Add parsley, basil, oregano, sea salt, and shrimp; cook for 20 minutes. Top with soy parmesan, if desired.

Dessert Drinks

These drinks are more than beverages. They are desserts in themselves, a refreshing, low-calorie way to satisfy the sweet tooth and top off any meal.

Strawberry Mint Cooler
Serves 2

2 cups apple juice
1 cup strawberries
1 teaspoon fresh mint, crushed

Blend and serve.

Lemon-Limeade
Serves 8

2 quarts (8 cups) water
½ cup fresh lemon juice
½ cup fresh lime juice
6 to 8 tablespoons honey

Combine all ingredients. Stir well and serve.

Peach Slush
Serves 2

1 cup ice
2 cups ripe peaches
2 teaspoons honey (or other sweetener)

Crush ice in a blender. Add peaches and honey and blend.

Desserts

Desserts are the *pièce de résistance* of every meal. With a little substituting here and there, you really can have your cake and eat it, too. And you can serve and enjoy healthful ice cream, cookies, and pies to your heart's content.

Nondairy Vanilla Ice Cream *Serves 4*

1 pound soft tofu
½ cup almonds, blanched
¾ cup honey

2 teaspoons vanilla
2 teaspoons guar gum

Drain tofu and place in a food processor. Add almonds and blend well until smooth. Combine honey and vanilla and mix again. Add guar gum and mix well. Pour into containers and place in freezer. Freeze until solid.

Molasses Cookies

Approx. 2 dozen

½ cup canola oil
½ cup honey
1 egg
½ cup blackstrap molasses
½ cup soy milk or nut milk
2½ cups rice flour

1 teaspoon baking soda
1 teaspoon cinnamon
1 teaspoon ginger
¼ teaspoon salt
1 cup raisins

Preheat oven to 350°F. Mix canola oil and honey. Combine with egg, molasses, and nondairy milk. Mix flour, baking soda, cinnamon, ginger, and salt. Combine all mixed ingredients and blend until batter is smooth. Add raisins and mix well. Drop batter onto a greased cookie sheet. Bake 12 minutes.

Soy milk can be purchased at a health food store. Alternatively, you can make your own nut milk. (See Almond Milk recipe.)

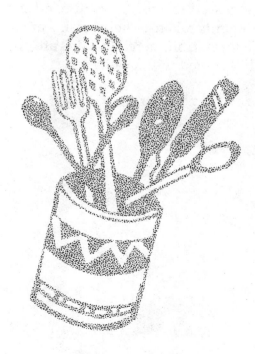

Molasses Raisin Bars

6 tablespoons canola oil
⅓ cup honey
⅔ cup blackstrap molasses
1 egg
1 teaspoon vanilla
1 cup rice flour

⅛ teaspoon salt
⅛ teaspoon baking soda
1 teaspoon cinnamon
⅛ teaspoon allspice
½ teaspoon ginger
½ cup raisins

Preheat oven to 375°F. Mix canola oil and honey. Combine with molasses, egg, and vanilla and blend well. Mix flour, salt, baking soda, cinnamon, allspice, and ginger. Combine all mixed ingredients until batter is smooth. Add raisins to batter and blend well. Pour batter into a well-greased 12x18 inch rectangular cake pan (other shapes may be used). Bake for approximately 17 minutes or until center is spongy and cakelike. Cut into bars when cool.

Note: For all dessert recipes, I recommend the use of unsprayed organic raisins. These raisins are available in health food stores. Commercial raisins are among the fruits most heavily sprayed with pesticides.

Oatmeal Cookies

Approx. 2 dozen

½ cup canola oil
¼ cup honey
1 egg, slightly beaten
2 teaspoons vanilla
½ teaspoon salt

1 cup rice flour
¾ teaspoon baking powder
2 cups rolled oats
1 cup raisins

Preheat oven to 370°F. Mix canola oil and honey. Combine with egg, vanilla, and salt and blend. Mix flour, baking powder, rolled oats, and raisins with a fork. Combine all ingredients and mix. A few teaspoons of water may be added until dough is of proper consistency. Spoon onto greased cookie sheets and flatten each cookie slightly with a spoon. Bake 12 to 15 minutes.

Pound Cake

Serves 8

2½ cups rice flour
½ teaspoon baking soda
1½ teaspoons baking
  powder
½ teaspoon sea salt

½ cup corn oil
⅓ cup honey
1 teaspoon vanilla
2 eggs
1 cup nut or soy milk

Preheat oven to 350°F. Sift together flour, baking soda, baking powder, and salt. Combine corn oil, honey, and vanilla. Separate eggs. Beat yolks and add to honey and oil mixture. Slowly add sifted ingredients to egg mixture with the nut or soy milk. Beat egg whites until stiff peaks form and fold them into the dough. Place dough in a well-greased loaf pan and bake 30 to 40 minutes or until a knife inserted in center of cake is clean when removed.

Applesauce Loaf

1½ cups rice flour
½ cup wheat germ
½ teaspoon salt
½ teaspoon baking powder

½ teaspoon baking soda
⅓ cup honey
½ cup corn oil
½ cup applesauce

Preheat oven to 375°F. Combine dry ingredients in a bowl. Mix corn oil with honey. Add applesauce, mixing well. Combine all ingredients. Place in a well-greased loaf pan. Bake 30 to 45 minutes. Test with knife to see if loaf is done.

Tea Cookies

2½ cups rice flour
¼ teaspoon sea salt
1½ teaspoons baking
   powder

½ cup corn oil
½ teaspoon vanilla
¼ cup honey
¼ cup water

Preheat oven to 325°F. Sift dry ingredients together. Combine corn oil with vanilla, honey, and ⅛ cup water. Combine the wet and dry ingredients, adding the rest of the water. Knead the dough into a ball, adding the rest of the water, as needed, to achieve a firm texture. Chill the dough for 1 hour and roll it to ¾ inch thick. Cut to desired shapes with a knife or cookie cutter. Transfer to greased cookie sheets and bake for 5 minutes.

Variations: Cookies may be varied by substituting orange juice for water or by adding ½ cup crushed almonds, walnuts, raisins, or poppy seeds.

Pie Crust Dough

Makes 1 crust (double to make 2)

1½ cups barley flour
½ cup wheat germ
1 teaspoon sea salt

½ teaspoon cinnamon
½ cup corn oil
4 tablespoons water

Preheat oven to 400°F. Combine dry ingredients in a bowl. Mix the corn oil into dry ingredients, using your fingers or a fork to break it into little pieces. Form the dough into a ball with your hands, adding water as needed. Refrigerate for 20 minutes. Roll the pie dough to the size of your pie pan, and then place in pie pan. Bake 8 to 10 minutes or until crust is golden brown.

Apple Pie

Serves 8

Pie Crust Dough recipe, double

4 to 5 apples, chopped
2 teaspoons cinnamon
pinch sea salt
2 tablespoons arrowroot
   powder

½ cup apple juice
1 egg yolk

Make Pie Crust Dough and divide into two equal pieces. Roll out one piece for bottom crust and place in oiled pie pan. Cover the other piece with a damp towel. Combine fruit, cinnamon, and sea salt. Set aside. Dissolve arrowroot powder in apple juice. Stir until they are well combined. (You may want to heat the mixture.) Pour arrowroot mixture over fruit and blend well. Let sit for a few minutes. Place filling in pie pan. Roll out top crust. Cover fruit mixture with crust. Prick crust with fork and glaze with egg yolk. Bake at 350°F for 30 minutes or until fruit is soft.

Blackberry Cream Pie   *Serves 8*

Pie Crust Dough recipe, single

2 cups blackberries (or strawberries, raspberries, blueberries,
    or boysenberries)
⅓ to ½ cup honey
1½ cups Nondairy Vanilla Ice Cream (page 344)

Make a single recipe of Pie Crust Dough. Line pie pan with the
dough and bake for 10 to 12 minutes. Combine berries and
honey until well-mixed. Place berries in pie pan and cover
with Nondairy Vanilla Ice Cream.

Baked Bananas   *Serves 4*

4 bananas
1 tablespoon lemon juice
2 tablespoons honey

Peel and slice bananas in half lengthwise. Place halves in a
well-oiled baking dish. Sprinkle with lemon juice and drizzle
with honey. Place in cold oven set to 400°F. When juice begins
to bubble, turn off heat. Leave in oven to finish baking on
retained heat.

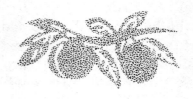

Persimmon Banana Treat

Serves 4

4 bananas
3 persimmons, ripe

2 tablespoons honey
½ cup coconut

Remove skin of persimmons and mash. Peel and slice bananas very thin. In each serving dish, alternate layers of banana and persimmon. Sprinkle with honey and cover with fine coconut. Chill and serve.

Banana and Sesame Butter

Serves 2

2 bananas, ripe
3 tablespoons raw sesame butter
½ teaspoon honey

Mash bananas in bowl and slowly blend in raw sesame butter and honey. This makes a highly nutritious dessert for women.

Apple-Banana Custard

Serves 2

4 ounces soft tofu
1 apple, red Delicious

1 banana, ripened
1 teaspoon honey

Combine tofu, apple, banana, and honey in blender and mix until a custardlike consistency is achieved.

Raspberry Cornmeal Cake

Serves 8

2 cups cornmeal
½ cup whole wheat pastry
  flour
1 teaspoon baking powder
½ teaspoon baking soda

1¼ teaspoon sea salt
1 egg, beaten
2 cups nondairy milk, vanilla
3½ tablespoons honey
2 tablespoons canola oil

Preheat oven to 425°F. Combine cornmeal, whole wheat flour, baking powder, baking soda, and sea salt in a mixing bowl. Combine egg, nondairy milk, honey, and canola oil. Mix all ingredients together and blend until batter is smooth. Pour into an oiled square cake pan and bake for 30 to 35 minutes or until knife comes out clean up on testing. Top with Raspberry Purée (see below).

Raspberry Purée

Serves 8

2 cups raspberries, fresh or frozen
½ cup honey

Purée in a food processor until smooth. Top cornmeal cake with this fruit treat before serving.

Bibliography

Books

Bernat, I. "Iron Deficiency." *Iron Metabolism:* New York: Plenum Press, 1983.

—. "Pyridoxine Responsive Anemia." *Iron Metabolism.* New York: Plenum Press, 1983.

Castleman, M. *The Healing Herbs.* Emmaus, PA: Rodale Press, 1991.

Colbin, A. *Food and Healing.* New York: Ballantine Books, 1986.

Erasmus, U. *Fats and Oils.* Burnaby, BC, Canada: Alive Books, 1986.

Gittleman, A. L. *Supernutrition for Women.* New York: Bantam Books, 1991.

Hasslering, B., S. Greenwood, M.D., and M. Castleman. *The Medical Self-Care Book of Women's Health.* New York: Doubleday, 1987.

Hogladaroom, G., R. McCorkle, and N. Woods. *The Complete Book of Women's Health.* Englewood Cliff, NJ: Prentice Hall, 1982.

Hylton, W. *The Rodale Herb Book.* Emmaus, PA: Rodale Press, 1974.

Kirschmann, J., and L. Dunne. *Nutrition Almanac.* New York: McGraw-Hill, 1984.

Kutsky, R. *Vitamins and Hormones.* New York: Van Nostrand Reinhold, 1973.

Lambert-Lagace, L. *The Nutrition Challenge for Women.* Palo Alto, CA: Bull Publishing Co., 1990.

Lark, S., M.D. *Anemia and Heavy Menstrual Flow. A Self-Help Program.* Los Altos, CA: Westchester Publishing Co., 1993.

—. *Anxiety and Stress: A Self-Help Program.* Los Altos, CA: Westchester Publishing Co., 1993.

—. *Chronic Fatigue and Tiredness: A Self-Help Program.* Los Altos, CA: Westchester Publishing Co., 1993.

—. *Fibroid Tumors and Endometriosis. A Self-Help Program.* Los Altos, CA: Westchester Publishing Co., 1993.

—. *Menstrual Cramps, A Self-Help Program.* Los Altos, CA: Westchester Publishing Co., 1992.

—. *Menopause Self Help Book.* Berkeley, CA: Celestial Arts, 1990.

—. *Premenstrual Syndrome Self Help Book.* Berkeley, CA: Celestial Arts, 1984.

—. *The Estrogen Decision.* Los Altos, CA: Westchester Publishing Co., 1994.

Lust, J. *The Herb Book.* New York: Bantam, 1974.

McDougall, J., and M. McDougall. *The McDougall Plan.* Clinton, NJ: New Win Publishing Co., 1983.

Mowrey, D. *The Scientific Validation of Herbal Medicine.* New Canaan, CT: Keats Publishing, 1986.

Murray, M. *The 21st Century Herbal Volume I.* Bellevue, WA: Vita-Line, 1985.

—. *The 21st Century Herbal Volume II.* Bellevue, WA: Vita-Line, 1985.

Padus, E. *The Woman's Encyclopedia of Health and Natural Healing.* Emmaus, PA: Rodale Press, 1981.

Rector-Page, L. *How to be Your Own Herbal Pharmacist.* Linda Rector-Page, 1991.

Reuben, C., and J. Priestly. *Essential Supplement for Women.* New York: Perigree Books, 1988.

Articles

Chapters 1, 2: Foods for Healthy Women and Foods to Avoid

Abraham, G. E. "Magnesium Deficiency in Premenstrual Tension." *Magnesium Bulletin* (1982): 1:68-73.

—. "Nutritional Factors in the Etiology of the Premenstrual Syndrome." *Journal of Reproductive Medicine* (1983): 28:446–64.

—. "Premenstrual Tension." *Problems in Obstetrics and Gynecology* (1980): 3(12):1-39.

Barale, R., et al. "Vegetables Inhibit, in Vivo, the Mutagenicity of Nitrite Combined with Nitrosable Compounds." *Mutation Research* (1983): 120:145.

Boulenger, J. P., et al. "Increased Sensitivity to Caffeine in Patients with Panic Disorders: Preliminary Evidence." *Archives of General Psychiatry* (1984): 41:1067–71.

Bristol, J. B. "Sugar, Fat, and the Risk of Colorectal Cancer." *British Medical Journal* (1985): 291:1457.

Bristol, J. B., et al. "Colorectal Cancer and Diet: A Case-Control Study with Special References to Dietary Fibre and Sugar." *Proceedings of the American Association of Cancer Research* (1985): 26:206.

Bruce, M., and M. Lader. "Caffeine Abstention in the Management of Anxiety Disorders." *Psychological Medicine* (1989): 19:211–14.

Charney, D. S., et al. "Increased Anxiogenic Effects of Caffeine in Panic Disorders." *Archives of General Psychiatry* (1985): 42:233–43.

Christensen, L. "Psychological Distress and Diet—Effects of Sucrose and Caffeine." *Journal of Applied Nutrition* (1988): 40(1):44–50.

Cremer, D. W., et al. "Dietary Animal Fat in Relation to Ovarian Cancer Risk." *Obstetrics and Gynecology* (1984): 63(6):88388.

Dalvit-McPhillips, S. "A Dietary Approach to Bulimia Treatment." *Physiology and Behavior* (1984): 33(5):769–75.

Dennefors, B. L., et al. "Progesterone and Adenosine 3',5'-monophosphate Formation by Isolated Human Corpora Lutea of Different Ages: Influence of Human Chorionic Gonadotrophin and Prostaglandins." *Journal of Clinical Endocrinology and Metabolism* (1943): 3:227-34.

DePirro, R., et al. "Insulin Receptors During the Menstrual Cycle in Normal Women." *Journal of Clinical Endocrinology and Metabolism* (1978): 46(6):1387-89.

Enig, M. G., et al. "Dietary Fat and Cancer Trends." *Federal Proceedings* (1978): 37:2215-20.

Erickson, K. L., and I. K. Thomas. "The Role of Dietary Fat in Mammary Tumorigenesis." *Food Technology* (1985): 69-73.

Ferrannini, E., et al. "Sodium Elevates the Plasma Response to Glucose Ingestion in Man." *Journal of Clinical Endocrinology and Metabolism* (1982): 54:455.

Freund, G. "Benzodiazepine Receptor Loss in Brains of Mice After Chronic Alcohol Consumption." *Life Sciences* (1980): 27(11):987–92.

Fullerton, D. T., et al. "Sugar, Opioids, and Binge Eating." *Brain Research Bulletin* (1985): 14(6):673–80.

Goei, G. S., et al. "Dietary Patterns of Patients with Premenstrual Tension." *Journal of Applied Nutrition* (1982): 34(1):4–11.

Goldin, B. R., and S. Gorbach. "The Effect of Milk and Lactobacillus Feeding on Human Intestinal Bacterial Enzyme Activity." *American Journal of Clinical Nutrition* (1984): 39:756-61.

———. "The Relationship Between Diet and Rat Fecal Bacterial Enzymes Implicated in Colon Cancer." *Journal of the National Cancer Institute* (1976): 57:371-75.

Goldin, B. R., et al. "Effect of Diet on Excretion of Estrogens in Pre- and Post-Menopausal Women." *Cancer Research* (1981): 41:3771-73.

———. "Estrogen Excretion Patterns and Plasma Levels in Vegetarian and Omnivorous Women." *New England Journal of Medicine* (1982): 307:1542-47.

Greenward, P. and E. Lanza. "Dietary Fiber and Colon Cancer." *Contemporary Nutrition* (1986): 11(1).

Hill, M. J., et al. "Gut Bacteria and Aetiology of Cancer of the Breast." *Lancet* (1971): 2:472-73.

Hoehn, S. K., and K. K. Carroll. "Effects of Dietary Carbohydrate on the Incidence of Mammary Tumors Induced in Rats by 7,12-Dimethylbenz(a)-Anthracene." *Nutrition and Cancer* (1979): 1(3):27-30.

Hollander, D., and A. Tarnawski. "Dietary Essential Fatty Acids and the Decline in Peptic Ulcer Disease." *Gut* (1986): 22(3).239.

Horrobin, D. F. "Essential Fatty Acid and Prostaglandin Metabolism in Sjogren's Syndrome; Systemic Sclerosis and Rheumatoid Arthritis." *Scandinavian Journal of Rheumatology Supplement* (1980): 61.242.

———. "Essential Fatty Acids and the Complications of Diabetes Mellitus." *Wien Klin Wochenschur* (1989): 101(8).289.

———. "Essential Fatty Acids in Clinical Dermatology." *Journal of the American Academy of Dermatology* (1987): 20(6).1045.

———. "The Regulation of Postaglandin Biosynthesis by the Manipulation of Essential Fatty Acid Metabolism." *Revue of Pure and Applied Pharmacologic Science* (1980): 4(4).339.

———. "The Role of Essential Fatty Acids and Prostaglandins in the Premenstrual Syndrome." *Journal of Reproductive Medicine* (1983): 28(7).465.

Horsman, A., et al. "Prospective Trial of Oestrogen and Calcium in Postmenopausal Women." *British Medical Journal* (1977): 2.789.

Howe, G. R., et al. "Dietary Factors and the Risk of Breast Cancer." Combined analysis of 12 case-controlled studies. *Journal of The National Cancer Institute* (1990): 82.561-69.

Hughes, R. E. "Hypothesis: A New Look at Dietary Fiber." *Human Nutrition: Clinical Nutrition* (1986): 40C:81-86.

Jones, D. V. "Influence of Dietary Fat on Self-Reported Menstrual Symptoms." *Physiology and Behavior* (1987): 40(4):483–87.

Kappas, A., et al. "Nutrition-Endocrine Interactions: Induction of Reciprocal Changes in the Delta-4-5-Alpha-Reduction of Testosterone and the Cytochrome p-450-Dependent Oxidation of Estradiol by Dietary Macronutrients in Man." *Proceedings of the National Academy of Science* (1983): 80:7646-49.

King, D. S. "Can Allergic Exposure Provoke Psychological Symptoms? A Double-Blind Test." *Biological Psychiatry* (1981): 16(1):3–19.

Kuchel, D., et al. "Catecholamine Excretion in Idiopathic Edema: Decreased Dopamine Excretion, a Pathologic Factor." *Journal of Endocrinology and Metabolism* (1977): 44:639.

Lee, M. A., et al. "Anxiety and Caffeine Consumption in People with Anxiety Disorders." *Psychiatry Research* (1985): 15:211–17.

———. "Anxiogenic Effects of Caffeine on Panic and Depressed Patients." *American Journal of Psychiatry* (1988): 145(5):632–35.

Levy, M., and E. Zylber-Katz. "Caffeine Metabolism and Coffee-Attributed Sleep Disturbances." *Clinical Pharmacology and Therapeutics* (1983): 33(6):770–75.

McDonald, R. H., et al. "Effects of Dopamine in Man: Augmentation of Sodium Excretion, Glomenrula Filtration Rate and Renal Plasma Flow." *Journal of Clinical Investigation* (1964) 43:1116.

McKeown, L. A., "Diet High in Fruits and Vegetables Linked to Lower Breast Cancer Risk." *Medical Tribune* (1992): 9:14.

Monteiro, M. G., et al. "Subjective Feelings of Anxiety in Young Men after Ethanol and Diazepam Infusions." *Journal of Clinical Psychiatry* (1990): 51(1):12–16.

Muggeo, M. et al. "Change in Affinity of Insulin Receptors Following Oral Glucose in Normal Adults." *Journal of Clinical Endocrinology and Metabolism* (1977): 44:1206-9.

Penrod, J. C., et al. "Impact on Iron Status of Introducing Cow's Milk in the Second Six Months of Life." *Journal of Pediatric Gastroenterology and Nutrition* (1990): 10:462-67.

Phillips, R. L. "Role of Life-Style and Dietary Habits Among Seventh-Day Adventists." *Cancer Research* (1975) 35:3513-22.

Porikos, K. P., and T. B. van Itallie. "Diet-Induced Changes in Serum Transaminase and Triglyceride Levels in Healthy Adult Men. Role of Sucrose and Excess Calories." *American Journal of Medicine* (1983): 75:624.

Rainey, J. M., Jr., et al. "Specificity of Lactate Infusion as a Model of Anxiety." *Psychopharmacology Bulletin* (1984): 20(1):45–9.

Rosenberg, I., et al. "Breast Cancer and Alcoholic Beverage Consumption." *Lancet* (1982): 1:267.

Rossignol, A. M. "Caffeine-Containing Beverages and Premenstrual Syndrome in Young Women." *American Journal of Public Health* (1985): 75(11):1335–37.

Rossignol, A. M., and H. Bonnlander. "Caffeine-containing Beverages, Total Fluid Consumption, and Premenstrual Syndrome." *American Journal of Public Health* (1990): 80(9):1106–10.

Rossignol, A. M., et al. "Tea and Premenstrual Syndrome in the People's Republic of China." *American Journal of Public Health* (1989): 79(1):67–69.

Sanders, L. R., et al. "Refined Carbohydrate as a Contributing Factor in Reactive Hypoglycemia." *Southern Medical Journal* (1982): 75:1072.

Seeley, S., and D. F. Horrobin. "Diet and Breast Cancer: The Possible Connection with Sugar Consumption." *Medical Hypothesis* (1978): 11(3):319-27.

Seelig, M. "Human Requirements of Magnesium: Factors that Increase Needs in Humans." Ed, J. Duriach. *International Symposium on Magnesium Deficiency in Human Pathology* (1971): 11.

Shirlow, M. J., and C. D. Mathers. "A Study of Caffeine Consumption and Symptoms: Indigestion, Palpitations, Tremors, Headache, and Insomnia." *International Journal of Epidemiology* (1985): 14(2):239–48.

Willet, W. D., et al. "Dietary Fat and the Risk of Breast Cancer." *New England Journal of Medicine* (1987): 316:22-28.

Wynder, E. L., and L.A. Cohen. "A Rationale for Dietary Intervention in the Treatment of Postmenopausal Breast Cancer Patients." *Nutrition and Cancer* (1982): 3(4):195-99.

Chapter 3: Premenstrual Syndrome (PMS)

Abraham, G. E., et al. "Effect of Vitamin B_6 on Plasma and Red Blood Cell Magnesium Levels in Premenopausal Women." *Annals of Clinical Laboratory Science* (1981): 11(4):333-36.

—. "Nutritional Factors in the Etiology of the Premenstrual Tension Syndromes." *Journal of Reproductive Medicine* (1983): 28(&):446-64.

—. "Premenstrual Tension." *Problems in Obstetrics & Gynecology;* (1980): 3(12):1-39.

Abraham, G. E., and J. T. Hargrove. "Effect of Vitamin B_6 on Premenstrual Symptomatology in Women with Premenstrual Tension Syndrome: A Double-Blind Cross-Over Study." *Infertility* (1980): 3:15565.

Argonz, J., and C. Albinzano. "Premenstrual Tension Treated with Vitamin A." *Journal of Clinical Endocrinology* (1950): 10:1579-89.

Barr, W. "Pyridoxine Supplements in the Premenstrual Syndrome." *Practitioner* (1984): 238:425-27.

Baumblatt, J. J., and F. Winston. Letter. "Pyridoxine and the Pill." *Lancet* (1970): 1:832.

Block, E. "The Use of Vitamin A in Premenstrual Tension." *Acta Obstetrics and Gynecology Scandinavia* (1960): 39:586-92.

Brush, M. G., and D. F. Horrobin. "Evening Primrose Oil in the Treatment of the Premenstrual Syndrome." Ed. *Clinical Uses of Essential Fatty Acids* (1982): 155-62.

Cunnane, S. C., and D. F Horrobin. "Parenteral Linoleic and Gammalinolenic Acids Ameliorate the Gross Effects of Zinc Deficiency." *Proceedings of the Society of Experimental Biology and Medicine* (1980): 164:583.

Curry, D. L., et al. "Magnesium Modulation of Glucose-Induced Insulin Secretion by the Perfused Rat Pancreas." *Endocrinology* (1977): 101:203.

Day, J. B. "Clinical Trials in Premenstrual Syndrome." *Current Medical Research Opinions* (1979): 6(Suppl. 5):40-45.

Facchinetti, F. "Oral Magnesium Successfully for Relieving Premenstrual Mood Changes." *Obstetrics and Gynecology* (1991): 78(2):177.

Gugliano, D., and R. Torrella. "Prostaglandin E1 Inhibits Glucose-Induced Insulin Secretion in Man." *Prostaglandins and Medicine* (1979): 48:302.

Horrobin, D. F. "A Biochemical Basis for Alcoholism and Alcohol-Induced Damage including the Fetal Alcohol Syndrome and Cirrhosis: Interferences with Essential Fatty Acid and Prostaglandin Metabolism." *Medical Hypotheses* (1980): 6(9):929.

—. "Essential Fatty Acids and the Complications of Diabetes Mellitus." *Wien Klin Wuchenschur* (1989): 101(8):289.

—. "The Regulation of Prostglandin Biosynthesis by the Manipulation of Essential Fatty Acid Metabolism." *Revue of Pure and Applied Pharmacology Science* (1980): 4(4):339.

—. "The Role of Essential Fatty Acids and Prostaglandins in the Premenstrual Syndrome." *Journal of Reproductive Medicine* (1983): 28(7):465.

Horton, R., and E. G. Biglier. "Effect of Aldosterone on the Metabolism of Magnesium." *Journal of Clinical Endocrinology* (1962): 22:1187.

Kerr, G. D. "The Management of the Premenstrual Syndrome." *Current Medical Research Opinions* (1977): 4(Suppl.4):29-34.

Kleine, H. O. "Vitamin A Therapie bei pra Menstruellen Nervosen Beschwerden." *Disch. med. Wschr.* (1954): 79:879-80.

Larsson, B., et al. "Evening Primrose Oil in the Treatment of Premenstrual Syndrome: A Pilot Study." *Current Therapeutic Research* (1989): 46:58.

London, R. "The Effect of a Nutritional Supplement on Premenstrual Symptomatology in Women with Premenstrual Syndrome." *Journal of the American College of Nutrition* (1991): 10(5):494.

London, R. S., et al. "The Effect of Alpha-Tocopherol O in Premenstrual Symtpomatology: a Double-Blind Trial." *Journal of the American College of Nutrition* (1983): 2:115-22.

Puolakka, J., et al. "Biochemical and Clinical Effects of Treating the Premenstrual Syndrome with Prostaglandin Synthesis Precursors." *Journal of Reproductive Medicine* (1985): 39(3):149-53.

Redmond, D. E., et al. "Menstrual Cycle and Ovarian Hormone Effects on Plasma and Platelet Monamine Oxidase (MAO) and Plasma Dopamine-Hydroxylase Activities in the Rhesus Monkey." *Psychosomatic Medicine* (1975): 37:417.

Richie, C. D, and R. Singkarmani. "Plasma Pyridoxal-5′-phosphate in Women with Premenstrual Syndrome." *Human Nutrition: Clinical Nutrition* (1986): 40C:75-80.

Simpson, L. O. "The Etiopathogenesis of Premenstrual Syndrome as a Consequence of Altered Blood Rheology: A New Hypothesis (evening primrose oil, fish oils)." *Medical Hypotheses* (1988): 25(4):189.

Williams, M. J., et al. "Controlled Trial of Pyridoxine in the Premenstrual Syndrome." *Journal of Internal Medicine Research* (1985): 13:174-79.

Chapter 4: Menstrual Cramps

Abraham, G. E. "Primary Dysmenorrhea." *Clinical Obstetrics and Gynecology* (1978): 21(1):139–45.

Bauer, U. "Six-Month Double-Blind Randomized Clinical Trial of Ginkgo Biloba Extract. Placebo in Two Parallel Groups in Patients Suffering from Peripheral Arterial Insufficiency." *Arzneim-Forsch* (1984): 34:716–21.

Butler, E. B., and E. McKnight. "Vitamin E in the Treatment of Primary Dysmenorrhoea." *Lancet* (1955): 1:844–47.

Fontana-Klaider, H., and B. Hogg. "Therapeutic Effects of Magnesium in Dysmenorrhea." *Schweiz Rundsch Med Prax* (1990): 17:79 (16):491–94.

Forman, A., U. Ulmsten, and K. E. Andersson. "Aspects of Inhibition of Myometrial Hyperactivity in Primary Dysmenorrhea." *Acta Obstet Gynecol Scand Suppl* (1983): 113:71–76.

Forster, H. B., H. Niklas, and S. Lutz. "Antispasmodic Effect of Some Medicinal Plants." *Planta Medica* (1980): 40:309–19.

Gebner, B., A. Voelp, and M. Klasser. "Study of the Long-term Action of a Ginkgo Biloba Extract on Vigilance and Mental Performance as Determined by Means of Quantitative Pharmaco-EEG and Psychometric Measurements." *Arzneim-Forsch* (1985): 35:1459–65.

Goodnight, S. H. "The Effects of Omega-3 Fatty Acids on Thrombosis and Atherogenesis." *Hematologic Pathology* (1989): 3(1):1.

Harada, M., M. Suzuki, and Y. Ozaki. "Effect of Japanese Angelica Root and Peony Root on Uterine Contraction in the Rabbit in Situ." *Journal of Pharm Dyn* (1984): 7:304–11.

Hazelhoff, B., T. M. Malingre, and D. K. Meijer. "Antispasmodic Effect of Valeriana Compounds: An In-Vivo and In-Vitro Study on the Guinea Pig Ileum." *Arch Int Pharmacodyn* (1982): 257:274–87.

Hikino, H. "Recent Research on Oriental Medicinal Plants." *Economic Medicinal Plant Research* (1985): 1:53–86.

Hindmarch, I., and Z. Subhan. "The Psychopharmacological Effects of Ginkgo Biloba Extract on Normal Healthy Volunteers." *International Journal of Clinical Pharmacology Research* (1984): 4:89–93.

Hollander, D., and A. Tarmawski. "Dietary Essential Fatty Acids and the Decline in Peptic Ulcer Disease." *Gut* (1986): 22(3):239.

Horrobin, D. F. "Essential Fatty Acids in Clinical Dermatology." *Journal of the American Academy of Dermatology* (1987): 20(6):1045.

——. "The Regulation of Prostaglandins in Biosynthesis by the Manipulation of Essential Fatty Acid Metabolism." *Revue of Pure and Applied Pharmacologic Science* (1980): 4(4):339.

Hudgins, A. P. "Vitamins P, C, and Niacin for Dysmenorrhea Therapy." *Western Journal of Surgery & Gynecology* (1954): 62:610–11.

Kryzhanovski, G. N., L. P. Bakuleva, N. L. Luzina, V. A. Vinogradov, and K. N. Iarygin. "Endogenous Opioid System in the Realization of the Analgesic Effect of Alpha-Tocopherol in Reference to Algomenorrhea." *Biull Eksp Biol Med* (1988): 105(2):148–150.

Kryzhanovski, G. N., N. L. Luzina, and K. N. Iarygin. "Alpha-Tocopherol Induced Activation of the Endogenous Opioid System." *Biull Eksp Biol Med* (1989): 108(11):566–67.

Luzina, N. L., and L. P. Vakuleva. "Use of an Antioxidant, Alpha-Tocopherol Acetate, in the Complex Treatment of Algomenorrhea." *Akush Ginekol* (Mosk) (1987): May(5):67–9.

Mieli-Fournial, A. "Trace Elements in the Treatment of Dysmenorrhea." *Biull Fed Soc Gynecol Obstet* (1968): 20(5):432–33.

Mowrey, D., and D. Clayson. "Motion Sickness, Ginger and Psychophysics." *Lancet* (1982): I:655–57.

Petkov, V. "Plants with Hypotensive, Antiatheromatous and Coronaroldilating Action." *American Journal of Clinical Medicine* (1979): 7:197–236.

Schaffler, V. K., and P. W. Reeh. "Double-Blind Study of the Hypoxia-Protective Effect of a Standardized Ginkgo Biloba Preparation after Repeated Administration in Healthy Volunteers." *Arzneim-Forsch* (1985): 35:1283–86.

Seifert, B., P. Wagler, S. Dartsch, U. Schmidt, and J. Nieder. "Magnesium—a New Therapeutic Alternative in Primary Dysmenorrhea." *Zentralbl Gynakol* (1989): 111(11):755–60.

Seltzer, S. "Pain Relief by Dietary Manipulation and Tryptophan Supplements." *Journal of Endodontics* (1985): 11:449–53.

Seltzer, S., D. Dewart, R. Pollack, and E. Jackson. "The Effects of Dietary Tryptophan on Chronic Maxillofacial Pain and Experimental Pain Tolerance." *Journal of Psychiatric Research* (1982): 17:181–86.

Shafer, N. "Iron in the Treatment of Dysmenorrhea: A Preliminary Report." *Current Therapy Research* (1965): 7:365–66.

Somerville, K. W., C. R. Richmond, and G. D. Bell. "Delayed Release Peppermint Oil Capsules (Colpermin) for the Spastic Colon Syndrome: A Pharmacokinetic Study." *British Journal of Clinical Pharmacology* (1984): 18:638–40.

Suekawa, M., A. Ishige, K. Yuasa, et al. "Pharmacological Studies on Ginger. I. Pharmacological Actions of Pungent Constituents (6)-Gingerol and (6)-Shogaol." *Journal of Pharm Dyn* (1984): 7:836–48.

Sung, C. P., A. P. Baker, D. A. Holden, et al. "Effects of Angelica Polymorpha on Reaginic Antibody Production." *Journal of Natural Products* (1982): 45:398–406.

Tanaka, S., Y. Ikeshiro, M. Tabata, and M. Konoshima. "Antinociceptive Substances from the Roots of Angelica Acutiloba." *Arzneim-Forsch* (1977): 27:2039–45.

Tanaka, S., Y. Kano, M. Tabata, and M. Konoshima. "Effects of Toki (Angelica Acutiloba Kitagawa) Extracts on Writhing and Capillary Permeability in Mice (Analgesic and Anti-Inflammatory Effects)." *Yakugaku Zassh* (1971): 91:1098–1104.

Yamahara, J., T. Yamada, H. Kimura, et al. "Biologically Active Principles of Crude Drugs. II. Anti-Allergic Principles in Shoseiryo-To Anti-Inflammatory Properties of Paeoniflorin and its Derivatives." *Journal of Pharm Dyn* (1982): 5:921–9.

Chapter 5: Endometriosis

Axelrod, A. E., A. C. Trakatellis. "Relationship of Pyridoxine to Immunological Phenomena." *Vitamins and Hormones* (1964): 22:591-607.

Baehner, R. I., L. A. Boxer. "Role of Membrane Vitamin E and Cytoplasmic Glutahione in the Regulation of Phagocytic Functions of Neutrophils and Monocytes." *American Journal of Pediatric Hematology and Oncology* (1979): 1(1):71-76.

Beisel, W. R. "Single Nutrients and Immunity." *American Journal of Clinical Nutrition* (1982): (suppl.) 35:417–68.

Biskind, M. S. "Nutritional Deficiency in the Etiology of Menorrhagia, Cystic Mastitis and Premenstrual Tension: Treatment with Vitamin B Complex." *Journal of Clinical Endocrinology and Metabolism* (1943): 3:227-34.

Biskind, M. S., and G. R. Biskind. "Effect of Vitamin B Complex Deficiency on Inactivation of Estrone in the Liver." *Endocrinology* (1942): 31:109-14.

Bondestam, M. et al. "Subclinical Trace Element Deficiency in Children with Undue Susceptibility to Infections." *Acta Paediatrica Scandinavica* (1985): 74 (4):515-20.

Butler, E. B., and E. McKnight. "Vitamin E in the Treatment of Primary Dysmenorrhoea." *Lancet* (1955): 1:844-47.

Chandra, R. K. "Trace Element Regulation of Immunity and Infection." *Journal of the American College of Nutrition* (1985): 4(1):5-16.

Cheng, E. W., et al. "Estrogenic Activity of Some Naturally Occurring Isoflavones." *Annals of New York Academy of Sciences* (1955): 61(3):652.

Cheraskin, E., et al. "Daily Vitamin C Consumption and Fatigability." *Journal of the American Geriatric Society* (1976): 24(3):136-37.

Clemetson, C. A. B., et al. "Capillary Strength and the Menstrual Cycle." *New York Academy of Sciences* (1962): 93 (7):277.

Cohen, J. D., and H. W. Rubin. "Functional Menorrhagia: Treatment with Bioflavonoids and Vitamin C." *Current Therapeutic Research* (1960): 2(11):539.

Das, U. N. "Antibiotic-Like Action of Essential Fatty Acids." *Journal of Canadian Medical Association* (1985): 132:1350.

Dickinson, L. F., et al. "Estrogen Profiles of Oriental and Caucasian Women in Hawaii." *New England Journal of Medicine* (1971): 291:1211-13.

Duchateau, J., et al. "Influence of Oral Zinc Supplementation on the Lymphocyte Response to Mitogens of Normal Subjects." *American Journal of Clinical Nutrition* (1981): 34:88–93.

Farley, P., M.D., and J. Foland, M.D. "Iron Deficiency Anemia: How to Diagnose and Correct." *Postgraduate Medicine* (1990): 87 (2):89-101.

Follingstad, A. R. "Commentary: Estriol the Forgotten Estrogen?" *Journal of the American Medical Association* (1978): 239 (1):29-30.

Fontana-Klaider, H., and B. Hogg. "Therapeutic Effects of Magnesium in Dysmenorrhea." *Schweiz Rundsch Med Prax* (1990): 17:79 (16):491-94.

Forster, H. B., H. Niklas, and S. Lutz. "Antispasmodic Effect of Some Medicinal Plants." *Planta Medica* (1980): 40:309-19.

Goldin, B. R., et al. "Effect of Diet on Excretion of Estrogens in Pre- and Post-Menopausal Women." *Cancer Research* (1981): 41:3771-73.

——. "Estrogen Excretion Patterns and Plasma Levels in Vegetarian and Omnivorous Women." *New England Journal of Medicine* (1982): 307:1542-47.

Gugliano, D., and R. Torella. "Protaglandin E_1 Inhibits Glucose-Induced Insulin Secretion in Man." *Prostaglandins and Medicine* (1979): 48:302.

Harris, C. "The Vicious Cycle of Anemia and Menorrhagia." *Canadian Medical Association Journal* (1957): 77:98.

Hikino, H. "Recent Research on Oriental Medicinal Plants." *Economic Medicinal Plant Research* (1985): 1:53-86.

Hodges, R. E, et al. "Hematopoietic Studies in Vitamin A Deficiency." *American Journal of Clinical Nutrition* (1978): 31:876-85.

Hudgins, A. P. "Vitamins P, C and Niacin for Dysmenorrhea Therapy." *Western Journal of Surgery and Gynecology* (1954): 62:610-11.

Hunt, J. R., et al. "Ascorbic Acid: Effect on Ongoing Iron Absorption and Status in Iron-Depleted Young Women." *American Journal of Clinical Nutrition* (1990): 51:649-55.

Kappas, A., et al. "Nutrition-Endocrine Interactions: Induction of Reciprocal Changes in the D^4 - 5a-Reduction of Testosterone and the Cytochrome p-450-Dependent Oxidation of Estradiol by Dietary Macronutrients in Man." *Proceedings of the National Academy of Sciences* (1983): 80:7646-49.

Kellis, T., and L. E. Vickery. "Inhibition of Human Estrogen Synthetase (Aromatase) by Flavones." *Science* (1984): 225:1032-34.

Kryzhanovski, G. N., et al. "Endogenous Opioid System in the Realization of the Analgesic Effect of Alpha-Tocopherol in Reference to Algomenorrhea." *Biull Eksp Biol Med* (1988): 105(2):148-50.

Kryzhanovski, G N., N. L. Luzina, and K. N. Iarygin. "Alpha-Tocopherol Induced Activation of the Endogenous Opioid System." *Biull Eksp Biol Med* (1989): 108(11):566-7.

Lithgow, P. M., and W. M. Politzer. "Vitamin A in the Treatment of Menorrhagia." *South African Medical Journal* (1977): 51:191.

Luzina, N. L., and L. P. Vakuleva. "Use of an Antioxidant, Alpha-Tocopherol Acetate, in the Complex Treatment of Algomenorrhea." *Akush Ginekol (Mosk)* (1987): May(5):67-69.

MacMahon, B., et al. "Urine Oestrogen Profiles of Asian and North American Women." *International Journal of Cancer* (1974): 4:161-67.

Mieli-Fournial, A. "Trace Elements in the Treatment of Dysmenorrhea." *Bulletin de la Federation des Societes de Gynecologic et d'Obstetrique de Langue Francaise* (1968): 20(5):432-33.

Chapter 6: Fibrocystic Breast Disease

Abrams, A. A. "Use of Vitamin E in Chronic Cystic Mastitis." *New England Journal of Medicine* (1965): 272:1080.

Aquino, T. I., and B. A. Eskin. "Rat Breast Structure in Altered Iodine Metabolism." *Archives of Pathology* (1972): 94:280.

Band, P. R., et al. "Treatment of Benign Breast Disease with Vitamin A." *Preventive Medicine* (1984): 13:549.

Eskin, E. A., et al. "Mammary Gland Dysplasia and Iodine Deficiency." *Journal of the American Medical Association* (1967); 200:115.

Krouse, T. B., et al. "Age-Related Changes Resembling Fibrocystic Disease in Iodine-Blocked Rat Breasts." *Archives of Pathology and Laboratory Medicine* (1979): 103:631.

London, R. S., et al. "Endocrine Parameters in Alpha-Tocopherol Therapy of Patients with Mammary Dysplasia." *Cancer Research* (1981):1:3811.

——. "Mammary Dysplasia: Clinical Response and Urinary Excretion of 11-Deoxy-17-Ketosteroids and Pregnanediol Following Alpha-tocopherol Therapy." *Breast* (1976): 4:19.

Mansel, R. E., et al. "The Use of Evening Primrose Oil in Mastalgia." *Clinical Uses of Essential Fatty Acids* (1983).

Simard, A. "Nutrition and Lifestyle Factors in Fibrocystic Disease and Cancer of the Breast." *Cancer Prevention and Nutrition* (1990): 567-72.

Soloman, D., et al. "Relationship Between Vitamin E and Urinary Excretion of Ketosteroid Fractions in Cystic Mastitis." *Annals of New York Academy of Science* (1972): 203:103.

Sundaram, G. S., et al. "Serum Hormones in Lipoproteins in Benign Breast Disease." *Cancer Research* (1981): 41:381.

Chapter 7: Anemia, Heavy Menstrual Flow, and Irregularity

Ajayi, O. A., et al. "Hematological Response to Supplements of Riboflavin and Ascorbic Acid in Nigerian Young Adults." *European Journal of Hematology* (1990): 44:209-12.

Beard, J. L., et al. "Impaired Thermoregulations and Thyroid Function in Iron-Deficiency Anemia." *American Journal of Clinical Nutrition* (1990): 52:813-19.

Brewer, G. J., et al. "Suppression of Irreversibly Sickled Erythrocytes by Zinc Therapy in Sickle Cell Anemia." *Journal of Laboratory and Clinical Medicine* (1977): 90(3):549-54.

Cheng, E. W., et al. "Estrogenic Activity of Some Naturally Occurring Isoflavones." *Annals of New York Academy of Sciences* (1955): 61(3):652.

Clemetson, C. A. B., et al. "Capillary Strength and the Menstrual Cycle." *New York Academy of Sciences* (1962): 93(7):277.

Cohen, J. D., and H. W. Rubin. "Functional Menorrhagia: Treatment with Bioflavonoids and Vitamin C." *Current Therapeutic Research* (1960): 2(11):539.

Corash, L., et al. "Reduced Chronic Hemolysis During High-Dose Vitamin E Administration in Mediterranean-Type Glucose-6-Phosphate Dehydrogenase Deficiency." *New England Journal of Medicine* (1980): 303:416-20.

Drake, J. R., and C. D. Fitch. "Status of Vitamin E as an Erythropoietic Factor." *American Journal of Clinical Nutrition* (1980): 33:2386-93.

Dunlap, W. M., et al. "Anemia and Neutropenia Caused by Copper Deficiency." *Annals of Internal Medicine* (1974): 80:470.

Farley, P., M.D., and J. Foland, M.D. "Iron Deficiency Anemia: How to Diagnose and Correct." *Postgraduate Medicine* (1990): 87(2):89-101.

Harris, C. "The Vicious Cycle of Anemia and Menorrhagia." *Canadian Medical Association Journal* (1957): 77:98.

Hines, J. D., and D. Love. "Abnormal Vitamin B_6 Metabolism in Sideroblastic Anemia: Effect of Pyridoxal Phosphate Therapy." *Clinical Research* (1975): 23:403A.

Hines, J. D., and J. W. Harris. "Pyridoxine-Responsive Anemia: Description of Three Patients with Megaloblastic Erythopoiesis." *American Journal of Clinical Nutrition* (1964): 14:137-46.

Hodges, R. E., et al. "Hematopoietic Studies in Vitamin A Deficiency." *American Journal of Clinical Nutrition* (1978): 31:876-85.

Hunt, J. R., et al. "Ascorbic Acid: Effect on Ongoing Iron Absorption and Status in Iron-Depleted Young Women." *American Journal of Clinical Nutrition* (1990): 51:649-55.

Jacobs, P., et al. "Gastric Acidity and Iron Absorption." *British Journal of Haematology* (1966): 12:728-36.

——. "Role of Hydrochloric Acid in Iron Absorption." *Journal of Applied Physiology* (1964): 19(2):187-88.

Kark, J. A., et al. "Pyridoxal Phosphate as an Antisickling Agent in Vitro." *Journal of Clinical Investigation* (1983): 71:1224.

Lane, M., and C. P. Alfrey, Jr. "The Anemia of Human Riboflavin Deficiency." *Blood* (1965): 25(4):432-42.

Leonard, P. J., and M. S. Losowsky. "Effect of Alpha-Tocopherol Administration on Red Cell Survival in Vitamin E-Deficient Human Subjects." *American Journal of Clinical Nutrition* (1971): 24:388-93.

Lithgow, P. M., and W. M. Politzer. "Vitamin A in the Treatment of Menorrhagia." *South African Medical Journal* (1977): 51:191.

Mangel, H., et al. "Thiamine-Dependent Beriberi in the Thiamine-Responsive Anemia Syndrome." *New England Journal of Medicine* (1984): 311:836-38.

McCurdy, P. R. "Is There an Anemia Responsive to Pantothenic Acid?" *Journal of American Geriatric Society* (1973): 21(2):88-91.

Mejia, L., and F. Chew. "Hematologic Effect of Supplementing Anemic Children with Vitamin A Alone and in Combination with Iron." *American Journal of Clinical Nutrition* (1988): 48:595-600.

Monsen, E. R. "Ascorbic Acid: An Enhancing Factor in Iron Absorption." *Nutritional Bioavailability of Iron*. American Chemical Society, (1982): 85-95.

Natta, C. L., and L. Machlin. "Plasma Levels of Tocopherol in Sickle Cell Anemia Subjects." *American Journal of Clinical Nutrition* (1979): 32:1359.

Natta, C. L., and R. D. Reynolds. "Apparent Vitamin B_6 Deficiency in Sickle Cell Anemia." *American Journal of Clinical Nutrition* (1984): 40:235-39.

Natta, C. L., et al. "A Decrease in Irreversibly Sickled Erythrocytes in Sickle Cell Anemia Patients Given Vitamin E." *American Journal of Clinical Nutrition* (1980): 33:968-71.

Niell, H. B., et al. "Zinc Metabolism in Sickle Cell Anemia." *Journal of the American Medical Association* (1979): 242 (24):2686-90.

Pearse, H. A., and J. D. Trisler. "A Rational Approach to the Treatment of Habitual Abortion and Menometorrhagia." *Clinical Medicine* (1957): 9:1081.

Pierce, L. E., and C. E. Rath. "Evidence for Folic Acid Deficiency in the Genesis of Anemic Sickle Cell Crisis." *Blood* (1962): 20:19.

Pope, G. S., et al. "Isolation of an Oestrogenic Isoflavone (Biochanin A) from Red Clover." *Chemistry and Industry* (1953): 10:1042.

Porter, K. G., et al. "Anemia and Low Serum Copper during Zinc Therapy." *Lancet* , (1977: 774).

Preuter, G. W. "A Treatment for Excessive Uterine Bleeding." *Applied Therapeutics* (1961): 5:351.

Rogers, L. E., et al. "Thiamine-Responsive Megaloblastic Anemia." *Journal of Pediatrics* (1969): 74(4):494-504.

Tant, D. "Megaloblastic Anemia due to Pyridoxine Deficiency Associated with Prolonged Ingestion of an Estrogen-containing Oral Contraceptive." *British Medical Journal* (1976): 979.

Taylor, F. A. "Habitual Abortion: Therapeutic Evaluation of Citrus Bioflavonoids." *Western Journal of Surgery, Obstetrics and Gynecology* (1956): 5:280.

Taymor, M. L., et al. "The Etiological Role of Chronic Iron Deficiency in Production of Menorrhagia." *Journal of the American Medical Association* (1964): 187:323.

——. "Menorrhagia due to Chronic Iron Deficiency." *Obstetrics and Gynecology* (1960): 16:571.

Viana, M. B., and R. I. Carvalho. "Thiamine-Responsive Megaloblastic Anemia Sensorineural Deafness and Diabetes Mellitus: A New Syndrome?" *Journal of Pediatrics* (1978): 93:235.

Williams, D. M. "Copper Deficiency in Humans." *Seminars in Hematology* (1983): 20(2):118-28.

Chapter 8: Fibroid Tumors

Biskind, M. S. "Nutritional Deficiency in the Etiology of Menorrhagia, Cystic Mastitis and Premenstrual Tension: Treatment with Vitamin B Complex." *Journal of Clinical Endocrinology and Metabolism* (1943): 3:227-34.

Biskind, M. S., and G. R. Biskind. "Effect of Vitamin B Complex Deficiency on Inactivation of Estrone in the Liver." *Endocrinology* (1942): 31:109-14.

Bulbrook, P. D., J. L. Haywar, C. Spicer. "Relationship between Urinary Androgen and Corticoid Excretion and Subsequent Breast Cancer." *Lancet* (1971): 2:395.

Butler, E. B., and E. McKnight. "Vitamin E in the Treatment of Primary Dysmenorrhoea." *Lancet* (1955): 1:844-47.

Cheng, E. W., et al. "Estrogenic Activity of Some Naturally Occurring Isoflavones." *Annals of New York Academy of Sciences* (1955): 61 (3):652.

Clemetson, C. A. B., et al. "Capillary Strength and the Menstrual Cycle.: *New York Academy of Sciences* (1962): 93 (7):277.

Cohen, J. D., and H. W. Rubin. "Functional Menorrhagia: Treatment with Bioflavonoids and Vitamin C." *Current Therapeutic Research* (1960): 2 (11):539.

Dickinson, L. F., et al. "Estrogen Profiles of Oriental and Caucasian Women in Hawaii." *New England Journal of Medicine* (1971): 291:1211-13.

Farley, P., M.D., and J. Foland, M.D. "Iron Deficiency Anemia: How to Diagnose and Correct." *Postgraduate Medicine* (1990): 87 (2):89-101.

Follingstad, A. R. "Commentary: Estriol, the Forgotten Estrogen?" *Journal of the American Medical Association* (1978): 239 (1):29-30.

Goldin, B. R., et al. "Effect of Diet on Excretion of Estrogens in Pre- and Post-Menopausal Women." *Cancer Research* (1981): 41:3771-73.

——. "Estrogen Excretion Patterns and Plasma Levels in Vegetarian and Omnivorous Women." *New England Journal of Medicine* (1982): 307:1542-47.

Harris, C. "The Vicious Cycle of Anemia and Menorrhagia." *Canadian Medical Association Journal* (1957): 77:98.

Hikino, H. "Recent Research on Oriental Medicinal Plants." *Economic Medicinal Plant Research* (1985): 1:53-86.

Hodges, R. E., et al. "Hematopoietic Studies in Vitamin A Deficiency." *American Journal of Clinical Nutrition* (1978): 31:876-85.

Hunt, J. R., et al. "Ascorbic Acid: Effect on Ongoing Iron Absorption and Status in Iron-Depleted Young Women." *American Journal of Clinical Nutrition* (1990): 51:649-55.

Kappas, A., et al. "Nutrition-Endocrine Interactions: Induction of Reciprocal Changes in the D^4 - 5a-Reduction of Testosterone and the Cytochrome p-450-Dependent Oxidation of Estradiol by Dietary Macronutrients in Man." *Proceedings of the National Academy of Sciences* (1983): 80:7646-49.

Kellis, T., and L. E. Vickery. "Inhibition of Human Estrogen Synthetase (Aromatase) by Flavones." *Science* (1984): 225:1032-34.

Kryzhanovski, G. N., et al. "Endogenous Opioid System in the Realization of the Analgesic Effect of Alpha-Tocopherol in Reference to Algomenorrhea." *Biull Eksp Biol Med* (1988): 105(2):148-50.

Kryzhanovski, G. N., N. L. Luzina, and K. N. Iarygin. "Alpha-Tocopherol Induced Activation of the Endogenous Opioid System." *Biull Eksp Biol Med* (1989): 108(11):566-67.

Lithgow, P. M., and W. M. Politzer. "Vitamin A in the Treatment of Menorrhagia." *South African Medical Journal* (1977): 51:191.

Luzina, N. L., L. P. Vakuleva. "Use of an Antioxidant, Alpha-Tocopherol Acetate, in the Complex Treatment of Algomenorrhea." *Akush Ginekol (Mosk)* (1987): May(5):67-69.

MacMahon, B., et al. "Urine Oestrogen Profiles of Asian and North American Women." *International Journal of Cancer* (1974): 4:161-67.

Monsen, E. R. "Ascorbic Acid: An Enhancing Factor in Iron Absorption." *Nutritional Bioavailablity of Iron.* American Chemical Society (1982): 85-95.

Pearse, H. A., and J. D. Trisler. "A Rational Approach to the Treatment of Habitual Abortion and Menometorrhagia." *Clinical Medicine* (1957): 9:1081.

Petkov, V. "Plants with Hypotensive, Antiatheromatous and Coronaroldilating Action." *American Journal of Clinical Medicine* (1979): 7:197-236.

Pope, G. S., et al. "Isolation of an Oestrogenic Isoflavone (Biochanin A) from Red Clover." *Chemistry & Industry* (1953): 10:1042.

Preuter, G. W. "A Treatment for Excessive Uterine Bleeding." *Applied Therapeutics* (1961): 5:351.

Roberts, H. J. "Perspective on Vitamin E as Therapy." *Journal of the American Medical Association* (1981): 246:129.

Shafer, N. "Iron in the Treatment of Dysmenorrhea: A Preliminary Report." *Current Therapy Research* (1965): 7:365-66.

Taylor, F. A. "Habitual Abortion: Therapeutic Evaluation of Citrus Bioflavonoids." *Western Journal of Surgery, Obstetrics and Gynecology* (1956): 5:280.

Taymor, M. L., et al. "The Etiological Role of Chronic Iron Deficiency in Production of Menorrhagia." *Journal of the American Medical Association* (1964): 187:323.

—. "Menorrhagia Due to Chronic Iron Deficiency." *Obstetrics and Gynecology* (1960): 16:571.

Wilcox, G., et al. "Estrogen Effects of Plant Foods in Postmenopausal Women." *British Medical Journal* (1990): 301:905-6.

Chapters 9, 10: Menopause, Osteoporosis, Heart Disease, and Breast Cancer

Albanese, A. A., et al. "Effect of a Calcium Supplement on Serum Cholesterol, Calcium Phosphorus, and Bone Density of Normal, Healthy Elderly Females." *Nutrition Report International* (1973): 8.119.

—. "Effects of Calcium Supplements and Estrogen Replacement Therapy on Bone Loss of Postmenopausal Women." *Nutrition Report International* (1981): 24.404.

Ammon, H. P. T., and A. B. Muller. "Forskolin: From Ayurvedic Remedy to a Modern Agent." *Planta Medica* (1985): 51:473-77.

Anastasi, J., and M. Steiner. "Effect of Alpha-Tocopherol on Known Platelet Aggregation." *Division of Hematologic Research, The Memorial Hospital; Pawtucket and Brown University, RI* (1974).

Ant, M. "Diabetic Vulvovaginitis Treated with Vitamin E Suppositories." *American Journal of Obstetrics and Gynecology* (1954): 67.407.

Baranov, A. I. "Medicinal Uses of Ginseng and Related Plants in the Soviet Union: Recent Trends in the Soviet Literature." *Journal of Ethnopharmacology* (1982): 6:339-53.

Bargallo Sangiorgi, G., et al. "Serum Potassium Level, Red Blood Cell Potassium and Alterations of Repolarization Phase of EKG in Old Subjects." *European Congress of Clinical Gerontology* (1983).

Baulbrook, P. D., et al. "Relationship Between Urinary Androgen and Corticoid Excretion and Subsequent Breast Cancer." *Lancet* (1971) 2:395.

Bierenbaum, M. L., et al. "Long Term Human Studies on the Lipid Effects of Oral Calcium." *Lipids* (1971): 7.202.

Biskind, M. S., and G. R. Biskind. "Effect of Vitamin B Complex Deficiency on Inactivation of Estrone in the Liver." *Endocrinology* (1942): 31.109.

Block, G. "Vitamin C and Cancer Prevention. The Epidemiologic Evidence. "*American Journal of Clinical Nutrition* (1991): 53.2701.

Block, M. T. "Vitamin E in the Treatment of Diseases of the Skin." *Clinical Medicine* (1953): 7.202.

Boykin, L. S. "Iron Deficiency Anemia in Postmenopausal Women." *Journal of the American Geriatrics Society* (1976): 24.558.

Brattstrom, L. E., et al. "Folic Acid Responsive Post-Menopausal Homocysteinemia." *Metabolism* (1985): 34.1073.

Breast Cancer Prevention Group. "Breast Cancer Environmental Factors." *Lancet* (1992): 340.904.

Butler, C. L., and C. H. Costello. "Pharmacologic Studies. I. Aletris Farinosa." *Journal of the American Pharmaceutical Society* (1944): 33:177-83.

Buttersworth, C. E., et al. "Improvement in Cervical Dysplasia Associated with Folic Acid Therapy in Users of Oral Contraceptives." *American Journal of Clinical Nutrition* (1982): 35.73.

Chang, J., et al. "Effect of Forskolin on Prostaglandine Synthesis by Mouse Resident Peritoneal Macrophages." *European Journal of Pharmacology* (1984): 103:303-12.

Cheng, E. W., et al. "Estrogenic Activity of some Naturally Occurring Isoflavones." *Annals of New York Academy of Sciences* (1955): 61(3).652.

Christy, C. J. "Vitamin E in Menopause: Preliminary Report of Experimental and Clinical Study." *American Journal of Obstetrics and Gynecology* (1945): 50.84.

Clemetson, C. A. B., et al. "Capillary Strength and the Menstrual Cycle." *New York Academy of Sciences* (1962): 93(7).277.

Cobb, J. O. "Demystifying Menopause." *The Canadian Nurse* (1987): 8.17.

Cohen, J. D., and H. W. Rubin. "Functional Menorrhagia: Treatment with Bioflavonoids and Vitamin C." *Current Therapeutic Research* (1960): 2(11).539.

Cohn, S. H., et al. "High-Calcium Diet and the Parameters of Calcium Metabolism in Osteoporosis." *The American Journal of Clinical Nutrition* (1968): 21.1246.

Cordova, C., et al. "Influence of Ascorbic Acid on Platelet Aggregation in Vitro and in Vivo." *Atherosclerosis* (1981): 41.15.

Corson, S. L., and V. G. Upton. "The Perimenopause: Physiologic Correlates and Clinical Management." *Journal of Reproductive Medicine* (1982): 27.1.

Cutick, R. "Special Needs of Perimenopausal and Menopausal Women." *Journal of Obstetric and Gynecologic Nursing* (1984): 3.685.

Dansi, A., et al. "The Estrogenic Activity of Polymerized Anol." *Biochimica e Terapia Sperimentale* (1937): 24:282-84.

Dawson-Hughes, B., et al. "A Controlled Trial of the Effect of Calcium Supplementation on Bone Density in Postmenopausal Women." *New England Journal of Medicine* (1990): 323 (13).878.

Dodds, E. C., and W. Lawson. "Estrogenic Activity of P-Hydroxypropenyl-Benzene (Anol)." *Nature* (1937): 139:1039.

——. "A Simple Oestrogenic Agent with an Activity of the Same Order as that of Oestrone." *Nature* (1937): 139:627.

Elghamry, M. I., and I. M. Shihata. "Biological Activity of Phytoestrogens." *Plantsa Medica* (1965): 13:352-57.

Faber, K. "The Dandelion-Taraxacum Officinale Weber." *Pharmazie* (1958): 13:423-35.

Finkler, R. S. "The Effect of Vitamin E in the Menopause." *Journal of Clinical Endocrinology* (1949): 9.89.

Formica, P. E. "The Housewife Syndrome: Treatment with the Potassium and Magnesium Salts of Aspartic Acid." Current Theraputic Research. 1962; 4.98.

Frithiof, et al. "The Relationship between Marginal Bone Loss and Serum Zinc Levels." *ACTA Med Scand* (1980): 27.67.

Fuchs, N. K. "Magnesium: The Key to Calcium Absorption." *Let's Live* (1985):

Gallagher, J. C., and B. L. Riggs. "Current Concepts in Nutrition: Nutrition and Bone Disease." *New England Journal of Medicine* (1978): 298.193.

Gallagher, J. C., et al. "Intestinal Calcium Absorption and Serum Vitamin D Metabolites in Normal Subjects and Osteoporotic Patients." *Journal of Clinical Investigation* (1979): 64.729.

Gerster, K. "Potential Role of Beta Carotene in the Prevention of Cardiovascular Disease." *International Journal of Vitamin and Nutrition Research* (1991): 61.277-91.

Gibson, M. R. "Glycyrrhiza in Old and New Perspectives." *Lloydia* (1978): 41:3348-54.

Goldin, B. R., et al. "Effect of Diet on Excretion of Estrogens in Pre-and Post-Menopausal Women." *Cancer Research* (1981): 41.3771.

—. "Estrogen Excretion Patterns and Plasma Levels in Vegetarian and Omnivorous Women." *New England Journal of Medicine* (1982): 307.1542.

Gomez, E. T., and C. W. Turner. "Effect of Anol and Dihydrotheelin on Mammogenic Activity of the Pituitary Gland of Rabbits." *Proceedings of the Society for Experimental Biology and Medicine* (1938): 39:140-42.

Goodnight, S. H. "Assessment of the Therapeutic Use of Omega-3 Fatty Acids in Vascular Disease and Thrombosis." *Chest* (1991): 102(4).3745.

—. "The Effects of Omega-3 Fatty Acids on Thrombosis and Atherogenesis." *Hematologic Pathology* (1989): 3(1).1.

Gozan, H. A. "The Use of Vitamin E in the Treatment of Menopause." *New York State Medical Journal* (1952): 15.1289.

Hahn, F. E., and J. Ciak. "Berberine." *Antibiotics* (1976): 3:577-88.

Hain, A. M., and J. C. B. Sym. "The Control of Menopausal Flushes by Vitamin E." *British Medical Journal* (1943): 7.9.

Hanset, A. E., et al. "Eczema and Essential Fatty Acids." *American Journal of Diseases of Children* (1947): 73.1.

Harris, C. "The Vicious Cycle of Anemia and Menorrhagia." *Canadian Medical Association Journal* (1957): 77.98.

Harrison, M., et al. "Calcium Metabolism in Osteoporosis." *Lancet* (1961): 5.1015.

Hasling, C., et al. "Calcium Metabolism in Postmenopausal Osteoporotic Women is Determined by Dietary Calcium and Coffee Intake." *Journal of Nutrition* (1991): 112.1119-1126.

Haspels, et al. "Disturbance of Tryptophan Metabolism and its Correction During Oestrogen Treatment in Postmenopausal Women." *Maturitas* (1978): 1.15.

—. "Estrogens and Vitamin B_6." *Frontiers of Hormone Research* (1975): 3.199.

Havsteen, B. "Flavonoids, a Class of Natural Products of High Pharmacological Potency." *Biochemical Pharmacology* (1983): 32:1141-8.

Hayakawa, R., et al. "Effects of Combination Treatment with Vitamin E and C on Chloasma-Pigmented Contact Dermatitis. A Double-Blind Control Clinical Trial." *ACTA Vitaminol Enzymol* (1981): 3n.s.(1).31.

Heaney, R. P., et al. "Effect of Calcium on Skeletal Development, Bone Loss, and Wrist Fractures." *The American Journal of Medicine* (1991): 5B: 23S-28S.

Hennekens, C. A., et al. "Beta Carotene and Cardiovascular Disease. Beyond Deficiency. New Views on the Functions and Health Effects of Vitamins." *New York Academy of Sciences* (1992): 22.

Henson, D. L., et al. "Ascorbic Acid. Biological Functions and Relation to Cancer." *Journal of the National Cancer Institute* (1991): 83(8).547-50.

Hill, M. J., et al. "Gut Bacteria and Aetiology of Cancer of the Breast." *Lancet* (1971): 2:472-73.

Hollander, D., and A. Tarmawski. "Dietary Essential Fatty Acids and the Decline in Peptic Ulcer Disease." *Gut* (1986): 22(3).239.

Horrobin, D. F. "Essential Fatty Acid and Prostaglandin Metabolism in Sjogren's Syndrome. Systemic Sclerosis and Rheumatoid Arthritis." *Scandinavian Journal of Rheumatology Supplement* (1980): 61.242.

—. "Essential Fatty Acids and the Complications of Diabetes Mellitus." *Wien Klin Wochenschur* (1989): 101(8).289.

—. "The Regulation of Prostaglandin Biosynthesis by the Manipulation of Essential Fatty Acid Metabolism." *Revue of Pure and Applied Pharmacologic Science* (1980): 4(4).339.

Horsman, A., et al. "Prospective Trial of Oestrogen and Calcium in Postmenopausal Women." *British Medical Journal* (1977): 2.789.

Howe, G. R., et al. "Dietary Factors and the Risk of Breast Cancer: Combined Analysis of 12 Case-Controlled Studies." *Journal of the National Cancer Institute* (1990): 82:561-69.

Hunter, D. T. "Antioxidant Micronutrients and Breast Cancer." *Journal of the American College of Nutrition* (1992): 11(5):633.

Jowsey, J. "Osteoporosis: Its Nature and the Role of Diet." *Postgraduate Medicine* (1976): 60(2).75.

Kavinovsky, N. R. "Vitamin E and the Control of Climacteric Symptoms." *Annals of Western Medicine and Surgery* (1950): 4(1).27.

Kellis, T., and L. E. Vickery. "Inhibition of Human Estrogen Synthetase (Aromatase) by Flavones." *Science* (1984): 225.1032-34.

Kruse, C. A. "Treatment of Fatigue with Aspartic Acid Salts." *Northwest Medicine* (1961): 6.597.

Kuhnau, J. "The Flavonoids: A Class of Semi-Essential Food Components: Their Role in Human Nutrition." *World Review of Nutrition and Diet* (1976): 24:117-91.

Leathwood, P. D., and F. Chauffard. "Aqueous Extract of Valerian Reduces Latency to Fall Asleep in Man." *Planta Medica* (1985): 54:144-48.

Leathwood, P.D., et al. "Aqueous Extract of Valerian Root (Valeriani Officinalis L.) Improves Sleep Quality in Man." *Pharmacol Biochem Behavior* (1982): 17:65-71.

Lee, C. J., et al. "Effects of Supplementation of the Diets with Calcium and Calcium-Rich Food on Bone Density of Elderly Females with Osteoporosis." *American Journal of Clinical Nutrition* (1981): 34.819.

Licato, A. "Effect of Supplemental Calcium on Serum and Urinary Calcium in Osteoporotic Patients." *Journal of the American College of Nutrition* (1992): 11(2). 164-67.

Lindquist, O. "Influence of the Menopause on Ischemic Heart Disease and its Risk Factors and on Bone Mineral Content." *ACTA Obstetrica et Gynecologica Scandinavica* (1982): 110.7.

Lutz, J. "Calcium Balance and Acid Base Status of Women as Affected by Increased Protein Intake and by Sodium Bicarbonate Ingestion." *American Journal of Clinical Nutrition* (1984): 39.20.

Machtey, I., and L. Ouaknine. "Tocopherol in Osteoarthritis: A Controlled Pilot Study." *Journal of the American Geriatrics Society* (1978): 26.328.

Manku, M. S., et al. "Prolactin and Zinc Effects on Rat Vascular Activity: Possible Relationship to Dihomogammalinolenic Acid and to Prostaglandin Synthesis." *Endocrinology* (1979): 104.774.

Manson, T., et al. "A Prospective Study of Vitamin C and the Incidence of Coronary Heart Disease in Women." *Circulation* (1992): 85.865.

Marcus, R. "The Relationship of Dietary Calcium to Maintenance of Skeletal Integrity of Man. An Interface of Endocrinology and Nutrition." *Metabolism* (1982): 31.93.

Marshall, D. H., and B. E. C. Nordin. "The Effects of 1-Hydroxyvitamin D_3 with and without Oestrogens on Calcium Balance in Postmenopausal Women." *Clinical Endocrinology* (1977): 7.1595.

Marshall, D. H., et al. "The Prevention and Management of Postmenopausal Osteoporosis." *ACTA Obstet Gynecol Second suppl* (1977): 565-49.

Mattill, H. A. "Vitamin E." *Journal of the American Medical Association* (1938): 110.1831.

McLaren, H. C. "Vitamin E in the Menopause." *British Medical Journal* (1949): 12.1378.

Middleton, E. "The Flavonoids." *Trends in Pharmaceutical Science* (1984): 5:335-38.

Neuringer, M., and W. E. Connor. "Omega-3 Fatty Acids in the Brain and Retina; Evidence for their Essentiality." *Nutrition Review* (1986): 44(9).285.

Nicholson, J. P., and C. M. Resnick. "Outpatient Therapy of Essential Hypertension with Dietary Calcium Supplementation." *Journal of the American College of Cardiology* (1984): 2.616.

Nordin, B. E. G. "Clinical Significance and Pathogenesis of Osteoporosis." *British Medical Journal* (1971): 1.571.

Osilesi, O., et al. "Blood Pressure and Plasma Lipids during Ascorbic Acid Supplementation to Borderline Hypertensive and Normotensive Adults." *Nutrition Research* (1991): 11.405-12.

Pauling, L. "How Vitamin C can Prevent Heart Attack and Stroke." *Linus Pauling Institute of Science and Medicine Newsletter* (1992): 3.

Pauling, L. "Prevention and Treatment of Heart Disease. New Research Focus at the Linus Pauling Institute." *Linus Pauling Institute of Science and Medicine Newsletter* (1992): 1.

Pauling, L. "Vitamin C and Heart Disease: a Chronology." *Linus Pauling Institute of Science and Medicine Newsletter* (1992): 2.

Pope, G. S., et al. "Isolation of Oestrogenic Isoflavone (Biochanin A) from Red Clover." *Chemistry and Industry* (1953): 10.1042.

Potischman, N. "Association Between Breast Cancer, Plasma Triglycerides, and Cholesterol." *Nutrition and Cancer* (1991): 15:205-15.

Renaud, S., and L. McGregor. "Essential Fatty Acids and the Platelet Membrane in Relation to Aggregation." *Annales de la Nutrition et de l'Alimentation* (1980): 34(2). 265.

Riggs, L., et al. "Treatment of Primary Osteoporosis with Fluoride and Calcium. Clinical Tolerance and Fracture Occurrence." *Journal of the American Medical Association* (1987): 243.446.

Rude, R. K., et al. "Low Serum Concentrations of 1,25-Dihydroxyvitamin D in Human Magnesium Deficiency." *Journal of Clinical Endocrinology and Metabolism* (1985): 61.933.

Sabir, M., and N. Bhide. "Study of some Pharmacologic Actions of Berberine." *Indian Journal of Physical Pharmacology* (1971): 15:111-32.

Schrauzer, G. N., et al. "Selenium in the Blood of Japanese and American Women with and without Breast Cancer and Fibrocystic Disease." *Japanese Journal of Cancer Research* (1985): 76:374.

Schrauzer, G. N., and D. Ishmael. "Effect of Selenium and Arsenic on the Genesis of Spontaneous Mammary Tumors in Inbred C3H Mice." *Annals of Clinical and Laboratory Science* (1974): 4:441.

Schrauzer, G. N. "Selenium and Cancer: A Review." *Bioinorganic Chemistry* (1976): 5:275.

Schumann, E. "Newer Concepts of Blood Coagulation and Control of Hemmorhage." *American Journal of Obstetrics and Gynecology* (1939): 38:1002-7.

Schwartz, A. G. "Inhibition of Spontaneous Breast Cancer Formation in Female C3H-AVY/A Mice by Long-Term Treatment and Dehydroepiandrosterone." *Cancer Research* (1979): 39:1129.

Seelig, M. S. "The Requirements of Magnesium by the Normal Adult." *American Journal of Clinical Nutrition* (1964): 14.342.

Shute, E. V. "Notes on the Menopause." *Canadian Medical Association Journal* (1937): 10.350.

Shute, E. V., et al. "The Influence of Vitamin E on Vascular Disease." *Surgery, Gynecology and Obstetrics* (1948): 86.1.

Simin, T. "Vitamin C and Cardiovascular Disease. A Review." *The American College of Nutrition* (1992): 11(2).107-25.

Skrabel, F., et al. "Low-Sodium/High-Potassium Diet for Prevention of Hypertension. Probable Mechanisms of Action." *Lancet* (1981): 10.895.

Smith, C. J. "Nonhormonal Control of Vaso-Motor Flushing in Menopausal Patients." *Chicago Medicine* (1964): 67.193.

Stone, K. J., et al. "The Metabolism of Dihomogammalinolenic Acid in Man." *Lipids* (1979) 14.174.

Suekawa, M., et al. "Pharmacological Studies on Ginger. I. Pharmacological Actions of Pungent Constituents, (6) Gingerol and (6) Shogaol." *Journal of Pharmacologic Dynamics* (1984): 7:836-48.

Takeda, S. "Liquid Peroxidation in Human Breast Cancer Cells in Response to Gammalinolenic Acid and Iron." *AntiCancer Research* (1992): 12:329-34.

Tee Khaw, K., and S. Thom. "Randomized Double-Blind Cross-Over Trial of Potassium on Blood Pressure in Normal Subjects." *Lancet* (1962): 9.1127.

Van Beresteijn, E. "Habitual Dietary Calcium Intake and Cortical Bone Loss in Perimenopausal Women: a Longitudinal study." *Calcified Tissue International* (1990): 47.338-44.

Vang, D. Y., and M. Herrian. "Plasma Dehydroepiandrosterone SO4 and Breast Cancer." *Acta Endocrinologica Supplementation* (1973): 177-30.

Vles, R. O. "Essential Fatty Acids in Cardiovascular Physiopathology." *Annales de la Nutrition et de l'Alimentation* (1980): 34(2).255.

Watson, E. M. "Clinical Experiences with Wheat Germ Oil (Vitamin E)." *Canadian Medical Association Journal* (1936): 2.134.

Weaver, C. M. "Calcium Bioavailability and its Relationship to Osteoporosis." *Proceedings for the Society of Experimental Biology and Medicine* (1992): 200.157-60.

Wertz, P. W., et al. "Essential Fatty Acids and Epidermal Integrity." *Archives of Dermatology* (1987): 123(10).1381.

Whitacre, F. E., and B. Barrera. "War Amenorrhea." *Journal of the American Medical Association* (1944): 124.399.

Wilcox, G., et al. "Estrogen Effects of Plant Foods in Post-Menopausal Women." *British Medical Journal* (1990): 301.905-6.

Zardize, D. G. "Fatty Acid Composition of Phospholipids in Erythrocyte Membranes and Risk of Breast Cancer." *International Journal of Cancer* (1990): 45:807-10.

Index

infertility and, 133
nutritional supplements
for, 134-38, 187-88
pain and, 133
phytoestrogens and, 137
symptoms, 132-33
Fish, 29-32
essential acids in, 29
iodine, vitamins, and
minerals in, 30
recipes, 338-40
sources of poly-
unsaturated fats, 29
storage, 31
Flax seed oil, 92
estrogen source, 26
Fluid retention
nutritional supplements
for, 95, 181
Folic acid, 124
Food
addictions, 183-85
caffeine content, 58
cravings, 89
digestive process and, 50
storage shortcuts, 209-10
toxic effects, 51
unfavorable types, 50-82
Formaldehyde in maple
syrup, 44
Fractures and osteoporosis,
155
Frequent urination in
menopause, 144
Fructose vs. sucrose, 44
Fruit, 32-37
calcium and, 35
handling for maximum
benefit, 36
magnesium and, 35
preparation, 202-4
selection, 199-201
as sugar substitute, 35
vitamins, minerals and,
32, 34-35
Fruit drinks, 246-47
Fruit juice
deficiencies relative to

whole fruit, 35
as sweetener, 44

GLA (gamma linolenic acid),
101
Gluten
allergy to, 14
in oats and rye, 15
Grains
cereals, 15-16
recipes, 304-5
storage, 17
types, 18
whole, 10-18
Gum recession and
osteoporosis, 155

Hair, nutritional supplements
for, 189-90
HDL (high density
lipoprotein), 161-62
Heart attack
anticlotting herbs and, 172
beta carotene and, 170
blood lipid profile and,
160
blood pressure and, 162
caffeine and, 56
cholesterol and, 161
diabetes and, 162
essential fatty acids and,
172
exercise and, 163
LDL/HDL ratio and, 162,
171
menopause and, 163-64
smoking and, 162
soybeans and, 21
stress and, 163
vitamins and, 171
Heart disease, 159-64
Heart palpitations in
menopause, 141
Heavy menstrual flow, 121-23
causes, 122
nutritional supplements
for, 123-29, 187-88

Height loss and osteoporosis,
155
Hematocrit, 119
Hepatitis and alcohol, 63
Herbal tea
menstrual cramps and,
104, 241
recipes, 237-43
Herbs, 45-46 See also specific
conditions or disease
cardiovascular disease,
172-73
diuretic, 95
relaxant/sedative, 93
sources, 45-46
stimulant, 94
High fiber diet
breast cysts and, 114
regulation of estrogen
levels, 11
High-density lipoprotein. See
HDL
Honey, 43
Hormone replacement
therapy. See HRT
Hormones and breast cysts,
113
Hors d'oeuvre recipes, 269-78
Hot flashes, 140-41
caffeine and, 55
nutritional supplements
for, 94, 152
tea for, 239
HRT (hormone replacement
therapy), 146
osteoporosis and, 158
Hypoglycemia, 179
Hypothyroidism, 179

Infertility, 133
Insomnia
magnesium and, 91
nutritional supplements
for, 93, 240
tea for, 240
Insulin balance, 67
Intercourse, painful in

menopause, 142
Intestinal gas and wheat
intolerance, 14
Iodine
breast cysts and, 116
sources, 30, 40
Iron
heme vs. nonheme, 127
herbs containing, 129, 138
for menstrual bleeding,
126
menstrual cramps and,
101
RDA, 101
sources, 101, 120, 127, 195
Irregular menstrual bleeding,
121-23
nutritional supplements
for, 123-29
Irritability
in menopause, 144
PMS and, 87-88
Itching, 144

Kelp, 116
Kidney stones, 169
vitamin C and, 148

LDL (low density
lipoprotein), 33, 161
LDL/HDL ratio, 162, 171
Legumes, 18-24
common, 23-24
fiber in, 18-19
minerals in, 19
Leiomyoma. See fibroid
tumors
Lignans, 10
breast cancer and, 175
Low-density lipoprotein. See
LDL
Lunch meals, 233

Magnesium, 90-91
anxiety and, 91

depression and, 87-88
irritability and, 87-88
magnesium and, 90
mood swings and, 87-88
nutritional supplements
    for, 93-95, 179-80
stress and, 87
sugar imbalances and, 66
symptoms, 85
tea, 238
Ponstel, 97
Postum, 57, 213
Potassium
    fruits and, 34
    sources, 194-95
Potassium/sodium balance,
    35, 74
Potato
    benefits, 40
    recipes, 305-9
Poultry, 29-32
    essential acids, 29
    most healthful parts, 30
    preparation, 205-7
    selection, 205-7
    storage, 31
    types, 32
Premenstrual spotting and
    endometriosis, 106
Prostaglandin E. *See* PGE
Prostaglandins and essential
    fatty acids, 25
Provera, 122
Provitamin A, 87

Race and osteoporosis, 156
RDA (recommended daily
    allowance)
    calcium, 100, 168
    magnesium, 100
    phosphorus, 169
Recipes
    cereal, 252-60
    dessert, 341-52
    dip, 270-73, 294-95, 326
    fish, 338-40
    grain, 304-5

herbal tea, 237-43
hors d'oeuvre, 269-78
muffin, 261-63
pancake, 260-61
potato, 305-9
salad, 287-97
salad dressing, 298-301
sandwich, 302-4
sauce, 319, 324, 329-32
side dish, 307-10
snack, 268-78
soup, 279-87
spread, 264-66
starch, 305-6
tofu, 297
vegetable, 311-17
vegetarian main course,
    318-40
Rectal bleeding and
    endometriosis, 106
Red clover and breast cancer,
    174
Red meat, 74-80

Saccharin, 70
Salad
    dressing recipes, 298-301
    meals, 234-35
    mineral rich, 290, 295
    recipes, 287-97
    seafood, 293
Salt, 72-74
    breast cysts and, 113
    effects, 72, 75
    excess use, 73
    menopause and, 72
    substitutes, 73-74, 116, 218
Sandwich
    meals, 234
    recipes, 302-4
Saturated fat
    breast cysts and, 113
    digestive difficulty, 51
    effects, 74
    foods high in, 80
    obesity and, 76
Saturated oils and digestive

problems, 77
Saturated vs. unsaturated
    fats, 74
Sauce recipes, 319, 324, 329-32
Scaly skin and vitamin A, 147
Seafood
    meals, 236
    preparation, 205-7
    selection, 205-7
    storage, 31
    types, 32
Seed oils, uses, 28
Seeds, 24-29
    minerals in, 27
    nutrients in, 24, 26-27
    preferred in diet, 28
    selection and storage, 27,
        204-5
    uses, 27
    vitamins in, 26
Sexual desire, loss in
    menopause, 142-43
Side dish recipes, 307-10
Skin
    nutritional supplements
        for, 189-90
    yellowing and anemia, 119
Snack recipes, 268-78
Sodium/potassium balance,
    35, 74
Soup recipes, 279-87
Soybeans
    heart attacks and, 21
    regulation of estrogen, 11,
        19
Soyco, 22
Soymage, 22
Spices, 45-46
Spread recipes, 264-66
Starch
    benefits, 40
    recipes, 305-6
Stimulants, caffeine, 52
Stress
    essential fatty acids and, 92
    heart attack and, 163
    management in
        menopause, 146

PMS and, 87
vitamin C and, 89
Substitute products, 221
Substitutes for
    alcohol, 65, 214-15
    beef, 22
    butter, 216-17
    caffeine beverages, 57, 213
    chocolate, 43
    dairy products, 215-17
    high stress ingredients,
        219-20
    margarine, 82
    milk, 16, 247-51
    poultry, 217
    red meat, 217
    salt, 73-74, 116, 218
    sugar, 35, 43-45, 69-71, 214
    wheat, 15, 218
Sucrose vs. fructose, 44
Sugar, 66-71
    candida and, 68
    deleterious action, 66
    digestive difficulty, 51
    effects, 67
    food addiction and, 68
    insulin balance, 67
    menopause and, 68
    negative effects, 71
    PMS and, 66
    sources, 71
    substitutes, 43-45, 69-71,
        214
    uses, 66
Sweeteners, 42-46
    concentrated, 17
    fruit juice as, 44
    preferred, 43
Symptoms
    anemia, 118
    anxiety, 55
    bladder infections, 143
    dairy product allergies, 78
    dizziness, 100
    endometriosis, 106
    fibroid tumors, 132-33
    folic acid deficiency
        anemia, 124

About Susan M. Lark, M.D.

Susan M. Lark, M.D., is a noted authority on women's health care and preventative medicine. Dr. Lark has been on the clinical faculty of Stanford University Medical School, Division of Family and Community Medicine, where she continues to teach. She has been the director of a number of clinical programs for women and worked with thousands of patients in her twenty years of private practice. Dr. Lark lectures widely on women's health issues and is the author of a series of books published by Celestial Arts including: *PMS Self Help Book, The Menopause Self Help Book, Menstrual Cramps Self Help Book, Fibroid Tumors & Endometriosis Self Help Book, Heavy Menstrual Flow & Anemia Self Help Book, Anxiety & Stress Self Help Book, Chronic Fatigue Self Help Book, The Estrogen Decision Self Help Book, and The Women's Health Companion.* If you would like to contact her for more personalized guidance, Dr. Lark is available for phone consultation at (415) 964-7268. She Also presents workshops and seminars on women's health issues.